THE
CONSTIPATION
GAME PLAN

A **STEP-BY-STEP GUIDE** to Managing
Your Child's Chronic Constipation

Christine Stephenson, PT, DPT
www.constipationcoach.com

Constipation
Coach

The Constipation Game Plan: A Step-By-Step Guide to
Managing Your Child's Chronic Constipation
© 2022, Christine Stephenson, PT, DPT. All rights reserved.

Published by Pine Trail Books, Rapid City, SD

ISBN 979-8-9853536-0-0 (paperback)
ISBN 979-8-9853536-1-7 (eBook)
Library of Congress Control Number: 2022900526

This book is intended to provide accurate information with regard to its subject matter and reflects the opinion and perspective of the author. However, in times of rapid change, ensuring all information provided is entirely accurate and up-to-date at all times is not always possible. Therefore, the author and publisher accept no responsibility for inaccuracies or omissions and specifically disclaim any liability, loss or risk, personal, professional or otherwise, which may be incurred as a consequence, directly or indirectly, of the use and/or application of any of the contents of this book.

Publication managed by AuthorImprints.com

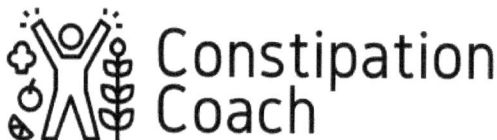

Constipation
Coach

www.constipationcoach.com

LEGAL DISCLAIMER

This book and the information provided in it are based on the author's personal experiences and detail the author's personal opinions about chronic constipation in children. The author is not your healthcare provider. Nothing in this book is intended to diagnose, treat, cure, or prevent any condition or disease. Please consult with your own physician or healthcare specialist regarding the suggestions and recommendations made in this book prior to implementing them, to ensure that they will not harm you.

The author does not warrant that the information accessible via this book is accurate, complete, or current. The author will not be liable for damages arising out of or in connection with the use of this book. This is a comprehensive limitation of liability that applies to all damages of any kind, including without limitation, compensatory, direct, indirect, or consequential damages; loss of data, income, or profit; loss of or damage to property or person; and claims of third parties. Use of this book implies your acceptance of these disclaimers and limitation of liability.

CONTENTS

WHY I WROTE THIS BOOK

C hronic constipation can be one of the most challenging situations to parent your way through. It can be heartbreaking: seeing your child in tears on the toilet because they know they need to poop but they can't and they know it's going to hurt if they do. It can be frustrating: having to pick up a sick kid from school for a stomachache, again, and then hearing the doctor say, again, that she is "just" constipated. It can be gross: getting poop streaks out of underwear is not a delightful chore.

Treating chronic constipation is also challenging. I know, because as a physical therapist I've been working with kids with urinary and fecal incontinence for the last nine years. For reasons that I will get into in Chapter 1, these kids almost always are constipated to some degree. Many have severe constipation and have had it for years. I learned early in my career that if I was going to successfully treat incontinence, I was going to have to learn how to treat constipation.

So what does a physical therapist (PT) do for constipation? We teach a child how to sit on the toilet, to use their abdominal muscles to bear down, and to relax their pelvic floor muscles when trying to push out poop. These are all important skills to master in order to control chronic constipation. Unfortunately, the discipline of PT doesn't have *all* the tools to manage this condition.

What I've come to realize, over the years, is that no single discipline can treat most cases of chronic constipation. Many disciplines can help: Physicians can prescribe medicines to make the stool soft and help it move through the system. Nutritionists can try to improve diet. Behavioral therapists can work on fear of toileting and on helping kids stick to a toileting schedule. Occupational therapists can help kids better recognize and respond to urges. But any one of these interventions, utilized in isolation, is not likely to be successful.

There's good news, though. Treating chronic constipation is not rocket science. It takes time and persistence. What I found with my chronically constipated kids is that I was using only about 50 percent of my time with them to do PT-related activities. Other parts of the session were spent discussing laxative use and clean-outs and how to get kids to drink more water and follow a toileting schedule. I had to explain the situation to school nurses and other adults and teach everyone how to manage the stress that accompanies this challenging condition.

As a PT, I feel pretty comfortable working with my kids in all of these areas. PTs work on *physical* aspects of health, but we are remiss if we don't acknowledge a mind-body connection in our patients and take a holistic, multi-disciplinary approach. Learning how to read and interpret research is an important part of a PT's education. So, I dove in and tried to teach myself everything about pediatric constipation.

What you will read in this book is a summary of what I have learned through research and working with hundreds of children and their families. Research into the digestive system is always evolving. This book contains a good round-up of what we currently know. Sometimes, there just isn't a good study backing up what I've learned in the clinic. I've tried hard to delineate in this book what is my clinical opinion, and what is based on research.

My goal is to help as many people learn what they need to know to manage chronic constipation in kids. My sincerest hope is that your child soon feels better, happier, and more energetic.

A NOTE TO READERS

My intention is to help children and families whose lives are significantly impacted by *severe* constipation. These kids have been to the doctor multiple times for this issue, they miss school due to stomach aches, they suffer from fecal and/or urinary incontinence. Many children have mild, occasional constipation; I don't want to cause parents of these children undue concern. The techniques in this book will certainly be helpful for addressing mild constipation, but please don't let this book create constipation stress where there wasn't any previously.

HOW TO READ THIS BOOK

My philosophy when it comes to treating constipation is that children and their parents are more successful when they know why they are constipated. I ask my families to become constipation detectives. That way, they can pick which interventions are going to be the most effective right away, and they can problem solve any issues that come up later during the course of treatment.

Chapter 1 is an overview of digestion and of the causes of constipation early in life. It's a little longer than the other chapters, but it will give you the background knowledge you need. The subsequent chapters are an action plan for getting better. Ideally, you'll have time to read this book all the way through, because each of the steps is important for long-term relief from constipation. If you are in a hurry, I recommend that you give Chapter 1 a close read, then skim the rest of the book to pick out which chapters are the most relevant to read next.

CHAPTER 1

WHAT IS CONSTIPATION?

Y ou're reading this book, which means you already know what constipation looks like in your child. But it's helpful to know how your doctor defines it, and why your child may not always get the help they need.

Physicians use the Rome criteria for diagnosing constipation. To qualify for a diagnosis, a person needs to have two or more of the following symptoms for at least six months:

- Less than three bowel movements per week
- Pain with defecation
- Lumpy or hard or large diameter stools
- Feeling of incomplete emptying or a blockage
- The need to use manual techniques to have a bowel movement.

It is important to note that the frequency of bowel movements—less than three per week— is only *one* of the criteria needed for diagnosis. I frequently see children who have bowel movements every day but are still quite constipated.

Once a diagnosis is made, physicians try to determine if the constipation is functional or organic. Organic constipation means that there is an underlying pathology that caused the constipation. This could be Hirschsprung's Disease, celiac disease, structural abnormalities of the bowel, or neurologic conditions. Children with organic constipation may benefit from much of the information in this book, but they also need focused medical management of the underlying condition.

Functional constipation means that there is no known physiological cause—the child entered into a cycle of constipation by withholding stool. According to the most recent Rome criteria, functional constipation in kids over the age of four can be diagnosed when they have two of the following symptoms for two months:

- Two or fewer bowel movements in the toilet per week
- At least one episode of fecal incontinence (encopresis) per week
- A history of withholding stools
- A history of hard or painful poops
- The presence of a large fecal mass in the rectum
- A history of large, hard stools, aka "toilet cloggers"

By a huge margin, most constipation in kids is functional constipation. A diagnosis of functional constipation can be super frustrating for families. While it is a relief to know that there is no disease process affecting your child, that doesn't mean the symptoms are any less serious or have less of an impact on your life. Too often, once organic

constipation is ruled out, parents are given a recommendation of a daily MiraLax dose and sent on their way. I once
had a GI doc tell me that these kids with functional constipation are just going to grow up to be adults with irritable
bowel syndrome. As if that is an adequate outcome!

Children with constipation deserve better than a life
with irritable bowel syndrome. Ask any adult with irritable
bowel syndrome, constipation prevalent. They are miser-
able! Chronic constipation is much easier to treat in children than it is in an adult. So let's dig deeper into how we
got here and what to do about it.

Before we can get into the detective work necessary to
figure out how to resolve your child's constipation, it's
important to understand how the GI tract works.

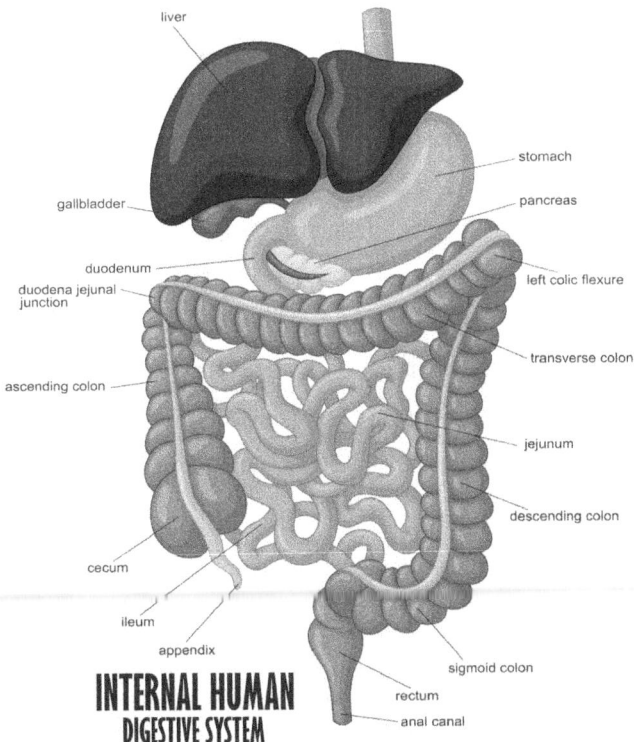

liver

stomach

pancreas

gallbladder

duodenum

left colic flexure

duodena jejunal
junction

transverse colon

ascending colon

jejunum

descending colon

cecum

ileum

appendix

sigmoid colon

INTERNAL HUMAN

rectum

DIGESTIVE SYSTEM

anal canal

The process of digestion, or turning food into energy and waste, starts with the chewing and mashing that happens in the mouth when we eat. If we eat slowly and chew well, we send a nice pureed lump of food into our stomach, where the food mixes with gastric juices to form a smooth soup.

Once the stomach soup is made, it passes from the stomach to the small intestine. The small intestine is a long, skinny tube that is all coiled up in the middle of the abdomen. It is here that the body takes all of the good stuff out of food (the vitamins and minerals, the fats and sugars, everything that helps us be the best us) and leaves what it doesn't need. By the time the digested food gets to the large intestine or colon, which is in the lower right side of your stomach, it is essentially diarrhea.

The large intestine, or colon, is a larger tube that goes up the right side of your abdomen, across under the lower rib cage, and down the left side of your abdomen. Its job is to remove some of the water from the waste that was produced in the small intestine. If everything is working correctly, the large intestine uses peristaltic contractions to push stool through the final stages of digestion (think of how you squeeze toothpaste up a toothpaste tube). Take a look at the Bristol Stool Scale, below. In a healthy person, the stool starts as type 7 (diarrhea) in the lower right part of the abdomen, and ends as type 4 (a soft, smooth sausage) in the rectum.

The Bristol Stool Form Scale

Type 1	Separate hard lumps, like nuts (hard to pass)
Type 2	Sausage-shaped but lumpy
Type 3	Like a sausage but with cracks on its surface
Type 4	Like a sausage or snake, smooth and soft
Type 5	Soft blobs with clear-cut edges (passed easily)
Type 6	Fluffy pieces with ragged edges, a mushy stool
Type 7	Watery, no solid pieces ENTIRELY LIQUID

The Bristol Stool Form Scale. Reproduced by kind permission of the late Dr K W Heaton, Formerly reader in Medicine at the University of Bristol. Reproduced as a service to the field of medical professionals by Norgine Ltd. ©2017 Norgine group of companies.   UK/COR/0118/0853. Date of preparation January 2018.

(The Bristol Stool Form Scale was developed in 1997 by Ken Heaton, MD. It is generally accepted as a reliable tool to indicate colonic transit, or the speed at which stool moves through the large intestine. Types 1 to 3 indicate slow colonic transit, and types 5 to 7 indicate fast transit. Most health care providers consider types 3, 4 and 5 to be healthy stools.)

The final stop for the digestion train is the rectum, the muscular pouch that collects stool. When the stool arrives, the rectum stretches, and the stretch sends a signal to the brain that it's time to head to the toilet. Once a person is on the toilet, the stool descends to the anus, and the pressure from the poop causes the internal anal sphincter to relax in preparation for letting the stool out. All that's left is for the individual to get to the toilet and relax the external anal sphincter, the main muscle that we have voluntary control of when it comes to defecation. Once the external anal sphincter relaxes, the muscles of the rectum contract to push the stool out. Done and done.

Functional constipation usually enters the scene at this very last moment: the brain gets a signal that stool is in the rectum, the rectum gets ready to push it out, the internal anal sphincter relaxes, and, for whatever reason, the child doesn't use the restroom. Those little bodies do whatever they can to make sure the external anal sphincter doesn't open: stand on their toes, clench their bottoms, lie on their back and arch to raise their butt off the floor.

The reason functional constipation is so tricky, and prevalent, in kids, is because once a little body decides to hold in stool, that stool doesn't go away. The body continues to take water out of the stool in the rectum, making it harder. The child continues to eat, producing more stool that backs up behind the larger ball. Eventually, when the rectum gets super full, the child will again feel the urge to have a bowel movement. Usually, by this time, once they feel the urge they have to go NOW. Often these poops are huge ones—the infamous toilet cloggers. Sometimes they are not: the child passes just enough hard stool to relieve some of the pressure. They can also be painful. Parents and kids breathe a sigh of relief once the child has had a bowel movement (BM): "glad that's over with!" But, usually, the constipation is not over.

Constipation is a terrible cycle in kids for several reasons:

First, if a child passes a hard ball of stool, it frequently hurts. It's common for kids to decide (consciously or not) that they don't want to do that again. So the next time they feel an urge, they withhold again, and another hard ball of stool forms.

Second, the rectum and colon really have to stretch to accommodate several days' worth of stool. Once the rectum stretches, it stops sending a signal to the brain that it's full of poop. I tell kids that it's like if I put a paperclip on their ear: they might feel it for a minute or two, but eventually they wouldn't feel that pinch, and they would forget that the paperclip is there. Suddenly, a child is no longer making a decision to withhold stool. They are holding stool because they actually don't feel its presence.

The third reason this cycle is difficult is that a fair number of kids with functional constipation develop what is known as pelvic floor muscle dyssynergia. As I explained above, in a typical person the muscles of the rectum and the abdomen contract to push out stool while at the same time the muscles of the pelvic floor relax to let it out. Kids who have a long history of withholding bowel movements can reach a point where they are actually tightening the pelvic floor muscles while they are trying to push out a poop, which means that one group of muscles (the pelvic floor muscles) are actually working against another group (the muscles of the rectum and abdomen).

Finally, a stretched-out colon and rectum don't do their jobs as well as their normal-sized counterparts. They work by stretching and then contracting, but once they've stretched too far, they don't contract as well. It's like when you blow up the same balloon and release the air a hundred times. The balloon gets stretched and floppy. This is what happens in the GI tract. Often those huge toilet-clogging BMs aren't even clearing out all of the old stool that the colon and rectum have accumulated. A fair amount of stool is gone, but old stool is still there and new stool just starts accumulating again. It can take months of very vigilant constipation management to get the colon and rectum to shrink back and start working like normal again. (It can take years for older children and adults.)

Side-note about urinary and fecal incontinence

Constipation, or, more specifically, a back-up of stool in the rectum, is the number one cause of urinary and fecal incontinence, including bed-wetting. Here's why:

The pelvis, which is the bony case for the rectum, bladder, and reproductive organs, is not super big. If the rectum gets stretched out and enlarged due to a back-up of stool, there simply isn't a whole lot of room for the bladder to stretch out and do its job of holding pee. Kids with chronic constipation are often using the bathroom frequently, wetting the bed, or waking up at night to use the bathroom simply because there's no room for that urine.

A ball of stool in the rectum causes urinary incontinence in other ways, as well. It can put pressure on the bladder and cause the nerves of the bladder to misfire (like the rectum, the bladder works by stretching to accommodate pee and then contracting when a person sits on the toilet and relaxes). The stool pressing on the outside of the bladder can cause the bladder to contract as if it's too full. Poop in the rectum can also put pressure on the urethra, the tube leading from the bladder to the outside of the body. The urethra narrows and the pee comes out like a trickle instead of a strong stream, despite the child feeling a strong urge. When this happens, kids don't always fully empty their bladder, which can lead to bedwetting or daytime incontinence.

Constipation is the primary cause of fecal incontinence or encopresis. As long as they continue eating, children with a huge back up of stool in the rectum continue to digest and make new poop. If there is too much hard stool blocking the way, the fresher, softer stool will wind its way around the old poop and leak out without the child knowing it's happening. Alternatively, a child may get the urge to have a bowel movement, but only when the rectum is very, very full. These kids will rush to the bathroom and just not make it in time. Finally, bowel movements that have been sitting in the rectum for a long time can be very sticky, stinky and hard to wipe. A normal, soft stool that comes out soon after it enters the rectum is usually easy to wipe. If a child has streaks in the underwear because they have trouble wiping, it is considered fecal incontinence and a strong sign of constipation.

What I've just described is nowhere near simple, and it is about as broad an overview as a person can give of the gastrointestinal tract. There is so much involved: nerves, voluntary muscles, involuntary muscles, hormones, gut bacteria, behavioral patterns—and so many places that disruption can occur. Miss a meal? Have to go on three rounds of antibiotics to clear up an ear infection? Forget to drink water all day? Go on a banana and peanut butter binge? Have a stressful morning and miss your daily urge to poop? The GI tract loves routine, and some GI tracts are particularly likely to make their owners pay if the routine gets off. These kids (and their parents) are the ones who end up seeing me.

Why Is This Happening?

So what's going on with your kid, specifically? It takes a little detective work to figure it out and knowing when it started is key.

My baby has *always* been constipated

Newborns who are constipated are almost always constipated for a reason other than diet and exercise. Most pediatricians are very good at ruling out organic causes of constipation like spina bifida, Hirschsprung's Disease, Celiac Disease, hypothyroidism, and cystic fibrosis. Frequently, once organic constipation is ruled out, physicians try to help parents manage the symptoms by recommending giving the infant small amounts of water or apple or prune juice in addition to formula or nursing. If that doesn't work, suppositories or MiraLax are often the next step.

Physicians and parents are often stumped by an infant's constipation when the major diseases, genetic conditions, and neurological causes are ruled out.

Some infants are constipated due to hypotonia, which means generally low muscle tone. These infants, if you hold them up above your head like an airplane, will just droop like a handkerchief. They often hate tummy time because lifting their head is much harder work than it is for other infants. The cause of hypotonia can be investigated to a certain extent with genetic testing. If the tests are negative, their hypotonia gets the label "idiopathic."

Kids with hypotonia get constipated because they move less and later than typical infants do, and movement helps the digestive tract work better, especially once the baby starts eating solid foods. These children also don't have the muscle tone in the abdominal wall to provide the external pressure needed to help the colon do its job of moving poop along. By the time I see them in the clinic, it's not immediately obvious that they had lower muscle tone as an infant. But when I assess their core strength, they are almost always weak.

Acid reflux is strongly linked to chronic constipation in infants and young children, but it's tricky to figure out which comes first, the constipation or the reflux. An infant with reflux experiences pain in their stomach and esophagus after eating. These infants frequently don't like sitting upright because the pressure worsens the reflux. They will push back on their highchair or fall backwards when placed in a sitting position on the floor. This pushing back changes the way the abdominal muscles and the pelvic floor work together to move stool through the colon, causing constipation.

On the other hand, the infant may have been constipated first and the build-up of stool pushed up on the stomach, essentially making it smaller. The smaller stomach holds less food, causing the child to extend back to get away from the pressure from all that food and poop in their belly.

Enlarged tonsils and adenoids are often associated with constipation. Although research has not definitively linked these two conditions, I would conservatively estimate that at a minimum half of my severely constipated patients have had tonsils and adenoids removed. This may be because infants who have to work very hard to breath often do so by tightening the belly muscles and the pelvic floor muscles. This gives them the stability they need to suck in air past the obstruction (the enlarged tonsils and adenoids) or through the smaller airways. The problem is, this constant tightening of the pelvic floor can cause the stool to get stuck—the child is trying so hard to stabilize their trunk that they can't relax enough to fully empty the rectum. They get constipated, the constipation leads to reflux, which often causes coughing, making it even harder to breath. The same process is in the works for kids with respiratory conditions such as reactive airway disease, asthma and sleep apnea.

My baby started getting constipated when we introduced foods

The introduction of solid foods is a frequent cause of constipation in young infants. This may be because the first foods we typically introduce in the United States are, by nature, constipating.

What are you supposed to give kids if they have diarrhea? The BRAT diet: bananas, rice, applesauce and toast. Do you know why? All of those foods are particularly good at plugging up the GI tract. Three of them are among the first foods that many parents give to infants. If your baby was slightly susceptible to constipation (for any of the reasons listed above), introducing processed white rice and bananas early in their food life may have been the proverbial straw that broke the camel's back. Most jarred baby food has cooked apples and pears as a base. While raw apples and pears often have a laxative effect, cooking them releases pectin, and the pectin can be constipating. So even though your child is getting fruits and vegetables, they can also be getting constipated.

Once babies start eating solids, we start to feed them "toddler food," and almost every processed food for toddlers is constipating. Goldfish crackers. Yogurt melts. Pureed fruit pouches. Cheerios. Mac and cheese. Simple sugars, complex carbohydrates, and very little fiber. We have all heard, as grownups, to shop the perimeter of the grocery store and avoid processed foods. But many babies and toddlers are given only processed foods, especially if they attend a daycare center. Even parents with the best of intentions can end up with a child who is constipated due to too much processed food.

Even if you managed to avoid all processed foods for your baby, your child may have a food sensitivity that leads to constipation. Food sensitivities are different from allergies, and testing for food sensitivities is not super reliable or supported by scientific evidence. But many people know that certain foods make their stomach hurt, give them gas, or cause constipation. The same goes for babies, but they don't have the ability to tell us when there is a causal link.

One common food sensitivity is to cow's milk. Cow's milk can be very constipating for certain people. Your child may not be allergic to milk or be lactose intolerant, but they could very well be sensitive to cow's milk in a way that other people are not. Eliminating dairy is a relatively easy way to test if it is contributing to constipation. (Please note, eliminating dairy is not the cure for chronic constipation, even if it was the cause. The stretched-out colon and rectum described above still need to be addressed.)

My toddler got constipated right around when we potty trained

Potty training can be a particularly fraught time! In my practice, I've identified two kinds of kids who are particularly likely to get constipated right around potty training time: first, the "parent pleasers." These children are so wonderful! They just want their parents to be proud of them. And their teachers to like them. And their babysitters to brag about them. And almost all of them were potty trained before the age of two. These are smart kids who were able to figure it out: if I pee in the toilet, people are so impressed!

My theory is that these children are able to learn quickly how to hold pee and poop, but they are too young to really understand the physical cues their body provides when they have an urge. So they hold and hold and hold, and when an adult tells them to go to the bathroom, they go. When they have been doing this well for a while, they get fewer prompts from adults to use the restroom. They end up unintentionally holding their pee and poop longer and longer. The longer that poop sits in the system, the harder it gets. The cycle of constipation begins. (As a side note, many of these early potty trainers are successful initially but struggle with pee leaks for longer than toddlers who are trained later when they are more developmentally mature.)

The second child who gets constipated right around potty training is the busy kid who just can't be bothered with toileting. Often these kids are potty trained later. They do fairly well with pee, but sitting to have a bowel movement is just too much time away from all the fun. Parents of these kids tell me "well, he never has an accident, but when he has to go poop, he has to go NOW." Urgency is a hallmark of my busiest patients.

My child got constipated when they started school

Those two-year-olds who were too busy to have a BM? They may have done OK when they were at home with a parent who could remind them to sit on a regular schedule. Or at a daycare where timed bathroom breaks were a part of the schedule and never skipped. But once these kids go to kindergarten, they can really get backed up. There is so much to do! Who has time to poop? Parents might not know their child is getting backed up until they are really backed up. Not that many parents are like me and ask their kids every day if they pooped, what kind of poop it was, and if they felt like they got everything out!

Busy kids aren't the only ones who get backed up when they're at school. School can be stressful! A child who is particularly sensitive to noise and a busy environment (like almost every kindergarten room I've been in) may have a GI tract that just freezes up during the school day. At home they may have had a perfect rhythm of going to the bathroom every day after breakfast during quiet play time, but the school environment totally throws off that rhythm, and they get backed up.

Other kids who get constipated at school frequently report that the bathrooms are gross. Or that they don't want other kids to hear them poop. Or the auto-flush function of the toilet scares them. Or that their teachers get mad when they ask to use the restroom and it's not a designated bathroom break time.

Side note on ADHD and constipation

Many of the kids I see with chronic constipation and fecal incontinence also have a diagnosis of ADHD. This relationship is backed up by a large study done in 2013 and published by the journal *Pediatrics*, the official journal of the American Academy of Pediatrics. The study reviewed the medical records of more than 700,000 kids whose parents were in the military and found that those with a diagnosis of ADHD were more than twice as likely as other children to see a doctor for constipation.

Researchers do not fully understand why ADHD might lead to constipation. ADHD is a neurological disorder, and there may be some impaired neurological function of the digestive organs that has yet to be identified. Children with ADHD may not receive the signal that stool has stretched the rectum, and therefore not void as frequently. There also is a behavioral component, as these children often tell me plainly that they will get an urge to have a BM but don't want to stop what they are doing to go to the toilet.

In addition, many of the medications used to treat ADHD are constipating. I had a psychiatrist tell me once that every prescription for ADHD should also come with a prescription for MiraLax. Intuniv, Ritalin, Strattera and Vyvanse all list constipation as possible side-effects. I do not recommend taking your child off these medications because they may be causing constipation, but knowing they cause constipation might help you better understand why your child is struggling.

Finally, it is well known in therapy circles that kids with ADHD can be pickier eaters than other kids. Picky eaters tend to prefer processed foods, which can easily get stuck in the system. These kids can also be grazers, meaning they eat small amounts all day long rather than sit calmly for a full meal. They eat quickly and hardly chew their food, which can slow digestion. Or their medications will suppress their appetite all day long and cause them to eat endlessly at dinnertime. Grazers miss out on an important reflex: the gastro-colic reflex. The stomach shrinks after a few hours of fasting between meals. When it is filled with food at a regular meal, the stretch of the stomach sends a signal to the colon to contract and move stool into the rectum. A small intake of food all day long means

that the stomach does not shrink and then stretch
to trigger this reflex.

My child was constipated, but that was years ago

So let's say you are a parent who noticed fairly early that
certain foods or drinks caused constipation in your child,
and you made the appropriate changes. Or your child got
constipated around potty training but eventually figured
things out and was able to have regular BMs on the toilet.
Done and done, right? Unfortunately, no. For all the reasons I described above (stretched out colon and rectum),
constipation can linger even after the cause has been
addressed. It's very likely that the constipation your child
has been struggling with for the last few months or years
has its roots in a constipation event that they had as a very
young child.

Side note on abdominal x-rays

Abdominal x-rays are sometimes used to help diagnose constipation. This is unfortunate, because
there is no evidence that x-rays are reliable at
diagnosing constipation or measuring its severity. Usually, a child gets an x-ray when their primary complaint for going to the clinic is abdominal
pain. The x-ray rules out any obstruction or foreign
object in the GI tract, that's all. Usually, no obstruction exists, and the parents get a report that there is
some amount of stool in the colon.

Even if x-rays were effective at diagnosing constipation, they usually don't provide an image of
the stool present in the rectum, which frequently

is what causes the most trouble in kids. The radiologist *can* measure rectal distension, which can help determine the severity of the back-up and maybe give an indication of how chronic a problem this is, but physicians don't always request that measurement. I have had plenty of kids with all the classic signs of constipation and an abdominal x-ray that says "normal." This is extremely misleading and unhelpful.

Let me be clear: if there is no suspicion of a structural problem, you shouldn't need an x-ray to diagnose constipation. Check out the Bristol stool scale again. Rabbit turds, lumps of grapes, and a log that looks cracked like the desert floor indicate constipation. Also, use the Rome criteria: do they feel as though there is poop there that they can't get out? Does it hurt to poop? Do they have huge poops or frequent diarrhea? Voila, constipation. There is no need to expose a child to radiation to answer these questions.

What Do We Do About It?

If your child struggles with any of the above symptoms, the first thing you should do is take a deep breath and give yourself, and your child, a break. So much of what leads to chronic, functional constipation in kids is not common knowledge. It is not taught in parenting classes and not part of the average well-baby visit. Somewhere along the line, your kid got constipated. It's nobody's fault.

The second thing you should do is have a conversation with your child discussing what you've learned so far. If your family has been dealing with this for years, it's likely you've made some mistakes, placing blame on yourself or your child for something that you didn't fully understand. So make an agreement with your child to wipe the slate clean and try a new approach together.

This book is intended to be a guide through a series of steps you can take to make progress in managing chronic constipation:

1) Have your child do a clean-out and find a daily medication routine that keeps stool soft and easy to pass.
2) Get your child on a toileting schedule.
3) Help your child learn how to sit on the toilet and understand how different muscles need to work to have a bowel movement.
4) Get moving: add a daily exercise routine designed to help promote bowel movements.
5) Identify and manage stress.
6) Make some changes to your child's diet that will help keep stool soft.
7) If necessary, find some professional help.

As I said earlier, in most cases there is no single cure for constipation. If that were the case, these kids would all be fine after starting a daily laxative. Some of the steps I recommend will be easy; others will require more time and effort, and there will be some children who need more intense interventions. It's important to understand that this process takes time. Usually kids start to see results pretty soon after implementing steps 1-3. The first three months are the most intense, then you will settle into an easier rhythm. Let's get started!

Side note on diet and exercise

If I hear one more person or read one more website claiming that diet and exercise can fix chronic constipation, I'm going to scream. I know from experience that diet and exercise alone can't fix chronic constipation. I suffered from chronic constipation through most of my 20s, a decade during which I ran frequently, carried a Nalgene bottle with me almost everywhere, and ate mostly vegetarian. If diet and exercise could fix constipation, I wouldn't have been constipated.

To be clear, diet and exercise play a part. Some research, almost all of it done on adults, suggests that adding a fiber supplement can help increase the frequency of bowel movements. And dehydration certainly pulls water out of stool out, making it harder and cracked. Fruits and vegetables soften the stool and push it along. And some exercises increase colonic motility, especially short, high-intensity interval sessions followed by rest. (Interestingly, long-duration moderate intensity aerobic exercise may contribute to constipation by decreasing blood flow and oxygen to the colon.) I will recommend some exercises and dietary changes for your kids. But I won't start, or stop, there.

What fixed my chronic constipation? First, recognizing it. For me, that meant learning that the urgent need I had to have a bowel movement 20 minutes into a run meant that I was backed up. Second, taking medication regularly. For the last ten years or so, I've taken about 300 mg of magnesium citrate at night. Do I wish I didn't have to? Sure. But having a daily medication to take is way better than going through cycles of constipation. Third, learning to pay attention to my body's schedule. If I don't have a BM after breakfast, I drink more water and eat some prunes and give myself several more times later in the day to sit and try again. It has taken years, and I'm still likely to get backed up quickly if I'm stressed out or not sleeping well or too busy to respond promptly to urges. I'll say it again: treating chronic constipation involves way more than just diet and exercise.

CHAPTER 1 TAKEAWAYS:

- Most kids with chronic constipation have *functional constipation*, which means they are voluntarily or involuntarily holding their stool.
- Chronic constipation in kids causes the rectum and colon to stretch, which means they do not do their jobs as well as they should.
- Laxatives will help a child with functional constipation start pooping again, but laxatives alone cannot break the cycle of chronic constipation.
- This book will help your child break the cycle of constipation with an approach that utilizes laxatives, a toileting schedule, changes to your child's posture on the toilet and the way they bear down, changes to diet, and stress management.

CHAPTER 2

FIRST STEP: MEDICATION
GET CLEANED OUT, AND FIND THE RIGHT DAILY LAXATIVE DOSE

A s a physical therapist and a generally pretty granola-y person, it pains me to say this: most people have to take laxatives daily to manage their constipation. Not for forever, but for a while. To successfully treat your child's constipation, you're going to have to give them medicine daily for the foreseeable future. Would you give your child medicine daily if they had high blood pressure? Diabetes? Allergies? Constipation is a medical condition that can be improved with the proper use of medication. Don't feel bad about it! You are not a failure as a parent because your child needs a daily laxative dose.

That cycle that I mentioned above? The one with the colon and rectum getting stretched out like an overused balloon, losing tone, losing mobility, and losing sensation? We can't break that cycle until the child does a clean-out to get all of the old stool out and then takes enough laxatives every day to keep their stool soft and moving along so it doesn't get backed up again.

The goal, with all of the interventions in this book, is to shrink the colon and rectum back to normal size so they are working again. Here's the thing: it is nearly impossible to do this with diet alone. You can make new stool softer by eating more fruits and vegetables—and you should!—but it is nearly impossible to eat enough produce consistently to keep a kid's colon clean. Kids are given junk food all day long when we are not around. Dr. Suess's birthday? Cookies! Class reward? Pizza party! Most kids don't have the willpower to resist that kind of temptation (neither do most adults, for that matter).

Laxatives are medicines that keep stool moving through your body. You're going to use laxatives in two ways: to get rid of old stool that is clogging and stretching out the colon and rectum (this is called a clean-out or disimpaction), and to keep the new stool soft and mobile so the colon and rectum have a chance to shrink back to their normal size (this is called a maintenance dose).

Laxatives come in primarily two varieties when used in children: stool softeners and stimulants.

Stool softeners, unsurprisingly, make the stool soft. Osmotic stool softeners do this by pulling water into the stool. Polyethylene glycol (MiraLax), magnesium citrate, milk of magnesia, sodium phosphate, and lactulose are osmotic laxatives. Docusate is a salt that also allows stool to absorb more water.

Stimulant laxatives include Bisacodyl (ExLax) and senna. These work by stimulating the colon to move stool along. For a long time, pediatricians did not like to prescribe stimulant laxatives to kids for fear that the bowel would become reliant on the stimulants. Research does not back up this assumption. And a bowel that has become stretched due to a back-up of stool often benefits from a stimulant laxative to move that softened stool along and tighten up the muscles of the colon.

What is a clean-out and how to do it

For most severely constipated kids, the first step of treatment is disimpaction. In laypeople terms, this means a bowel clean-out. In mild or moderately constipated kids, taking MiraLax for a few days in a row may be enough to get them pooping again and feeling better. But the long-term treatment of severe constipation is more effective if it starts with an aggressive clean-out, because a dose or two of a stool softener isn't sufficient to move out older, harder stool that has built up in the rectum and colon. You should work closely with your primary care provider to determine a safe, effective clean-out for your child. Here are the characteristics of the clean-outs that I have found to be the most effective in my patients:

- A high dose of polyethylene glycol (MiraLax) or magnesium citrate taken over a 2-3 day period,
- A stimulant laxative, taken once daily during the clean-out (senna or ExLax),
- Lots of fluid and maintaining a mostly-liquid diet for the duration of the clean-out.

The process ends when stool comes out looking like lemonade with little brown flecks in it. This process may be repeated every 4-6 weeks if it is an aggressive clean-out (gets to lemonade-like stool), and every two weeks if it is a gentler one (results in a lot of stool but no lemonade).

Your pediatrician or GI doctor might have a go-to clean out that they can recommend for your child. If not, several major hospital systems in the US publish recommendations for clean-outs on their websites—I've included my favorites in the references section at the end of the book.

I usually recommend that a child does a clean-out over a weekend or during a break from school when family outings will be minimal. If the child is young or suffering from fecal incontinence, I ask parents to let them wear a pull-up if the child wants to, although most of the time incontinence is not made worse during a clean-out. Your child's incontinence will get better eventually, but this first clean-out isn't about staying dry. It's about softening old stool and getting it out of the body. Make sure they are comfortable and aware of the larger goal.

Most pediatricians are coming around to the idea that clean-outs need to be fairly aggressive. When I started working with kids and asking my families to ask their pediatricians to guide them through a clean-out, it wasn't uncommon for pediatricians to recommend two caps of MiraLax for a few days in a row. Families would return to me in a week saying that their child has started pooping more and the poops were like "ribbons" or "worms." I'm always happy that a child is pooping more, but ribbon poops are a sign that the child is still backed up. The stool softener was effective at softening new stool, but the new soft stool is going around older, harder stool.

I frequently hear from families that the clean-out didn't work. Either, the child didn't have many BMs, they had watery diarrhea right away, or they had a lot of BMs but they didn't get to a clear yellow liquid with brown flecks in it. These circumstances are less common when a stimulant laxative is added to the regimen, but they do happen, and it's OK. The clean-out still did something, but it's likely it needs to be done a few more times. Ask your doctor if it's OK to do a clean-out once every 2-4 weeks. The amount of medicine and time needed to do the clean-out should decrease gradually as your child does more of them.

An important note about clean-outs: There's a reason I chose not to describe a specific clean-out in this book. While most pediatric GI clinics and societies recommend starting with disimpaction, there is very little research that indicates what type of clean-out is most effective. What will work for your child depends on so many things: the severity of their constipation, how much it impacts their lives and how willing they are to take medicines, what they have tried in the past and how it has worked, and your pediatrician's knowledge of your child's overall health and other conditions. I strongly recommend printing out one or more of the protocols referenced at the end of this book, bringing them to your pediatrician, and using them as a jumping off point to determine what is best for your child.

After the clean-out

Once you've found and implemented a clean-out regimen that works for your child, you need to figure out what your child's daily laxative dose should be. Remember, you may need to do clean-outs as often as every two weeks, at least initially. But it's important to keep your child's stool like soft-serve mashed potatoes, or a type 5 on the Bristol, between clean-outs. Some children may also need to take a daily stimulant laxative to help the colon shrink back to its normal size.

Kids often start with one capful of polyethylene glycol every evening. Smaller children may start at a half capful, and bigger kids often need two capfuls. Your doctor can recommend a dose based on your child's weight. Whatever the dose, most GI doctors recommend that a child take the entire dose in one sitting and drink it within 15 minutes. (Don't put two capfuls in the water bottle in the morning and have your child sip MiraLax all day long.) I find it is most effective to give the dose at night. The medicine works to soften the stool overnight. Then the child eats breakfast, does some exercises, elicits the gastrocolic reflex, and has a bowel movement before they leave for school.

Some children hate MiraLax. They can taste the supposedly tasteless powder in any liquid you mix it in. Or they don't like that it gives them gas. For these kids, ask your doctor about a daily magnesium citrate dose. Many kids like the product Natural Calm, which is a powder that comes in many palatable flavors. Some doctors prefer MiraLax because it stays almost entirely in the GI tract, whereas magnesium citrate is absorbed throughout the body. Even though magnesium citrate is available over-the-counter, you should ask your child's doctor if they have any concerns about using it.

If your child has been constipated for a long time and the stool softener alone isn't really doing the trick, you may want to ask your doctor about adding a stimulant laxative. Evidence shows that a stimulant laxative can speed the rebound of the colon and rectum, helping both to shrink back to a normal size more quickly than with just a stool softener. This is excellent news! It means you won't have to give as intense a dose of daily laxatives for as long.

If you decide to add senna or ExLax, you will want to experiment with the timing of the dose. Every child responds differently to stimulant laxatives. I've had kids who take an ExLax after school and have a BM after dinner, others who have the nurse give them a stimulant laxative at lunch so they have a BM before bed; and some who take it in the evening so they have a BM in the morning. When you find a time that works for your child, give the medicine at that time consistently. One thing to remember about the colon is that it likes regularity.

How long do I have to do the maintenance dose?
This is the million-dollar question, and the answer is: it depends. The goal for every intervention in this book is that the intensity and frequency of the intervention can be phased out as the colon and rectum shrink and start functioning the way they did before your child got constipated. How long this takes varies depending on the age of the child, how long they've been constipated and how severe it has been.

When it comes to laxatives, you should plan to keep your child on a maintenance dose, that is, one that keeps their poop around a type 5 on the Bristol, for months after their symptoms have resolved. Gradually, you can phase out the laxatives. Note that I did not say "stop the laxatives abruptly". According to the medical literature, everything I've recommended in this chapter is safe for kids. None of these medications will harm your child's GI tract in the long term. That said, your child's body *will* become reliant on these medications, and you should not stop them abruptly.

You're going to need to "down-train" your child's body so that they are no longer reliant on the medicines for normal bowel function. You will do this by gradually decreasing the daily dose. Again, please ask your pediatrician or GI doctor for guidance. You will know when to start weaning off laxatives because your child will have daily bowel movements and none of the secret signs of constipation (see below) for at least three months.

When to consider enemas

If your child is suffering from incontinence along with constipation, and the clean-outs don't seem to make a difference (or if the difference is short-lived), you may consider the Modified O'Regan Protocol, or MOP. The MOP provides guidance on using saline enemas daily, in conjunction with a daily polyethylene glycol dose, for several months to help break down and eventually pass an old, hard mass of stool in the rectum.

Saline enemas use a tube to stream saltwater into the rectum. The water stretches the rectum, and the salt pulls even more water into the rectum, helping to produce a forceful contraction. Saline enemas only work in the rectum and the last part of the colon, but they can effectively dislodge stubborn stool that other laxatives just can't budge.

Kids and families are often super nervous about the idea of an enema, but I've found that if the concept and the rationale are presented in a non-fearful way, many kids are game to give an enema a try. They're tired of incontinence, after all, and tired of doing clean-out after clean-out. After the first few enemas, kids often feel much better, and implementing the entire MOP protocol is no problem.

Many pediatricians bristle at this idea; they believe that enemas are too traumatic for children. Some GI docs feel the same way. I have heard GI doctors say that enemas teach a child to contract the pelvic floor muscles when these children really need to learn how to relax, that enemas further stretch an already-stretched rectum, and that children become dependent on enemas.

It's true that a child will be told to use their pelvic floor muscles to hold saline in when doing an enema. And it's true that, to be successful in the long-term, kids need to learn how to relax their pelvic floor muscles. But in my experience the kids who are undergoing the MOP have no regression in their pelvic floor muscle control as measured by the biofeedback that I use in the clinic. What's more, I often teach kids a contract/relax method for learning to relax the pelvic floor muscles: pull up and contract for as long as you can, then relax. This exercise teaches the muscles and nerves to know the difference between contraction and relaxation.

It's also true that a saline enema works in part by stretching the rectum. The saline itself stretches the rectum, and then the salt pulls even more water into the rectum. But this is for a few minutes at a time, not continuously for days and days. If we can't get the ball of stool out of the rectum, it will be stretched for months or even years.

Finally, children may become dependent on enemas. This is true. Children are going to become dependent on any form of laxative you give them. But it is possible to safely wean children off of enemas. "The MOP Book," by urologist Steve Hodges, MD, is a complete guide to implementing the MOP safely and with long-term success. I recommend bringing it to your doctor and discussing it as an option for your child.

Please note: do not try to give an enema to a child who is unwilling or who doesn't understand what you are doing. This would definitely be traumatic for a child and counter-productive. It also could be dangerous, as the enema tube could tear the anus. Just don't do it.

Also: there is a risk of dehydration with saline enemas. Make sure your pediatrician gives you the OK before starting the MOP. If your child receives an enema and you don't feel all the saline came out, contact your pediatrician.

CHAPTER 2 TAKEAWAYS:

- Laxatives are used to manage constipation in two ways: disimpaction, or removing a large amount of old stool that is blocking the way, and maintenance, or keeping new stool soft and moving.

- Work with your doctor on determining how to use medicines to give your child a clean-out. A few sample protocols are in the reference section of this book. Severely constipated kids often need several clean-outs before they achieve disimpaction.

- After successful disimpaction, or between clean-outs, give your child a maintenance laxative dose that helps them achieve a daily bowel movement that is the consistency of soft-serve ice cream.

- Plan to continue to give your child laxatives for several months after their symptoms improve, and do not stop the maintenance laxative dose cold turkey.

CHAPTER 3

YOUR NEW ROUTINE

Clean-out accomplished? Daily laxative dose established? Perfect. Now let's get into a GI-resetting routine.

I hope your child is feeling better after doing the clean-out. I frequently have parents tell me their kids are less grumpy and more energetic. They also report that their child now has an enormous appetite! This is great, because we are going to base this new routine on three square meals a day with few snacks in between.

I mentioned earlier the gastro-colic reflex. This is the reflex that tells the colon to move things along after you eat a meal. This reflex gets stronger the bigger the degree of stomach stretch. It's usually strongest after breakfast because this is when the stomach undergoes the biggest stretch after a 12-hour (or so) fast. It's strong after lunch and dinner, too, as long as there is little to no snacking between meals.

For the next few weeks, your child is going to sit on the toilet to try to have a poop 15 minutes after each meal. They don't have to sit for forever. Usually I ask kids to sit no more than 5 minutes. But they do have to sit quietly, take some deep breaths, and listen to their body. For a long time, your child's brain has been missing the signals coming from the gut that they have stool that needs to come out. They need to re-learn what this signal feels like, and they won't do that unless they slow down and pay attention.

I hear from parents quite a bit that this schedule is tough to stick to, especially on school days. This is a very reasonable complaint! But I'm going to ask you and your child to figure out a way to make it work. If your child doesn't take the time to sit, they won't "hear" the signals their body is sending them, and all that medicine that went into the clean-out will go to waste.

If three times a day is just impossible, make sitting after breakfast the top priority. Your child may have to wake up 15 minutes earlier, eat breakfast (add a cup of hot tea if you really want to cover all of your bases, as hot liquids can stimulate colonic motility), get dressed, brush teeth, do some exercises, and then sit on the toilet.

If you only have one bathroom in your house and there just isn't a way for your child to get five minutes of alone time on the toilet in the morning, you may have to get your child's school nurse involved. Once they know about your child's struggle, usually nurses and teachers and administrators are happy to help. After all, your child won't learn as well if they aren't feeling good. Some of the kids I've worked with have developed a schedule with the school and are allowed to come in five minutes early to use the bathroom before school starts.

Lunch is often the timed void that is the hardest to fit in. Here again, I suggest that you get your school administrators involved. Usually recess is after lunch, and usually it can be arranged that the recess monitor lets your child in five minutes early or the teacher allows your child to miss the first five minutes of afternoon classes. If your child just can't find a time to sit after lunch, then right after getting home from school is the next best option.

It's pretty important during these first few weeks that you keep a poop chart. Look at the next page for a basic design.

We're going to add other daily activities in the next few chapters, so you will want to personalize this chart with whatever you decide are the highest priorities for your child. It can seem tedious, but it's super helpful.

Why you should use a poop chart:

- Your child will learn their body's routine.
- You will be able to reward your child for doing the work.
- You will be able to show your child how they have improved, especially if they get frustrated or tired of the routine.
- You will have a record to show your physician as you work through which medicines to take and when repeat clean-outs are necessary.

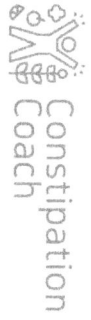

Constipation Coach

My Poop Chart

	Monday	Tuesday	Wednesday	Thursday	Friday	Saturday	Sunday
Sat After Breakfast							
Sat After Lunch							
Sat After Dinner							
Number of Poops, Size and Time of Day							

Please note: I don't think you should reward kids for *having* a BM. Instead, I'd like you to reward your child for *trying*. Sticking to this routine to break the constipation cycle is a lot of work, and it's not really your kid's fault that they have to do it. But they *do* have to do it. So give them a reward!

Examples of good rewards:

- A one-on-one outing with a parent, grandparent, or other cherished adult. If money is a challenge, kids love going to the park, on hikes, to public fountains, public concerts, or to the play area at the mall.
- A small piece of something your child collects: Legos, Calico Critters, Angry Birds, pencils, stickers, etc.
- For older kids, they can build up to bigger rewards with a token system, where they get a token for a chart filled out more than 80 percent and then 5 tokens equals a larger toy.
- Getting to choose the entire menu for a home-cooked meal.
- Getting to choose what to watch on family movie night or what game to play on game night.
- Getting to pick a parent to do a dreaded chore (cleaning their room, folding their laundry).

CHAPTER 3 TAKEAWAYS:

- Your child is most likely to poop after eating, so set up a toileting schedule that has them trying to poop after meals, whether they feel an urge or not.
- Use a chart to keep track of when your child sits and when they have bowel movements. This will help you figure out their patterns and will help your doctor advise you in laxative use.
- Reward your child for *trying* to have a BM, not for having one.

CHAPTER 4

SITTING FOR SUCCESS

U sually kids start to feel so much better after implementing the steps in chapters two and three. These next couple of chapters are where we will really step it up to the next level of long-term constipation management. Taking medicine and sitting on a schedule will help your child feel better, but if they don't learn how to sit, how to breath, and how to move to make their bodies work better, they may be taking a laxative and sitting on a schedule for years.

The very first thing to learn is "perfect pooping posture" or PPP. PPP may sound and seem silly, but it is key to voiding easily and completely. Throughout most of human history, we have squatted to poop. For obvious reasons, we don't squat over the toilet much these days. We need to modify our posture on the toilet to mimic a squat.

The thing about squatting is, it's the perfect position to poop! When we are standing, the puborectalis muscle loops around our lower colon, tightening it up, so that stool doesn't leak out when we are walking around. When we squat, that muscle goes on slack so there is no longer a kink in the colon and the stool can move into the rectum and—voila—come out quickly and easily as a poop.

Toilets are obviously wonderful, but the way we typically sit on a toilet only puts the puborectalis muscle on partial slack. So we have to push to get the poop through that ring-around-the-colon, and we often don't fully empty our bowels. Also, a lot of people round their low back and suck in their bellies when trying to have a bowel movement on the toilet. Sucking in the belly often makes it harder to poop.

What you'll need:

To achieve Perfect Potty Posture, your child is going to need a foot stool. My favorite is an adjustable stool from Squatty Potty. This lightweight plastic stool can be set at 7" or 9" high and it's easy to clean. It lives under your toilet, which is key. Any stool that needs to be hauled across the bathroom every time your child needs to use it won't be used. Typical bathroom stools won't work because they don't allow your child's feet and knees to be as far apart as they need to be, and they often aren't the right height. Please, incur this one expense and buy a Squatty Potty (or a knock-off that has a height of 9") for your kid.

Steps to Achieving PPP

1) *Camel and Cow*

Have your child get on their hands and knees and learn the "Camel" and "cow" yoga poses. The camel has an arched back like a camel's hump. The cow has a swayed belly. Your child can breathe in while making the camel's hump and out while making the cow's belly, or vice versa. You can place your hand on their low back and ask them to push their back up into your hand to make the camel's hump. Sometimes I'll also tell kids to imagine they have a tail, and they will tuck their tail between their legs when they do a camel's hump, then stick it in the air when they do a cow's belly.

Camel and Cow are yoga poses provide a nice set of verbal cues to kids for how their back should be positioned on the toilet. When paired with breathing, camel and cow increase blood flow to the colon, which can help the colon move stool along. They also draw your child's attention to his belly and back, which can be an area they have learned to ignore because of discomfort.

2) *Camel and Cow again—this time on a bench.*

Have your child sit on a bench or a low chair with their feet on the ground, knees apart (they can sit on their Squatty Potty for this training). Ask them to do camel and cow again while sitting. Again, cueing them to think about their tailbone, tucking it under for camel and sticking it back for cow, can be helpful. They can also put their hands on their hips to feel how their hips and pelvis rock forward and back with each movement.

Once they have this down, have them stop in cow so their tailbone is back and their low back is arched. Then tell them to tip their trunk forward and put their forearms on their legs right by their knees. Cueing them to keep the cow's belly is key: most of the time when kids put their forearms on their knees, they round out their lower back. We don't want that ... we want the back to stay relatively flat as they lean their trunk forward (see picture).

Since the knees are apart, there should be room between the legs for the belly to hang out. When we learn how to push out poop, it's going to be important that there is room for the belly to become big; this is why the knees need to be slightly wider than the hips.

3) Once your child has achieved Perfect Potty Posture on a bench, it's time to move into the bathroom. First, have them practice with their clothes on. They should be sitting on the front half of the toilet seat. Their feet and knees should be slightly wider than their hips. Younger kids should not try to put their feet on the footprints on the Squatty Potty. They would need to bring their knees together to do this, and we want knees apart.

4) If your child looks like they are getting it, then it's time for them to try it for real. I hope that your child lets you stay in the bathroom to give them feedback. Most of the kids I work with need a bit of practice with PPP, and it's most effective to help them when they are actually on the toilet, ready to try to poop.

Here are some of my friends of different ages in PPP. They are four, nine and eleven years old, and I they are all on the same toilet with the same size stool. If your kid tells you they think the stool is too big for them, you can show them these photos and remind them that the stool is actually intended for adult use. Note: the bigger the kid, the further the knees are in front of the toes.

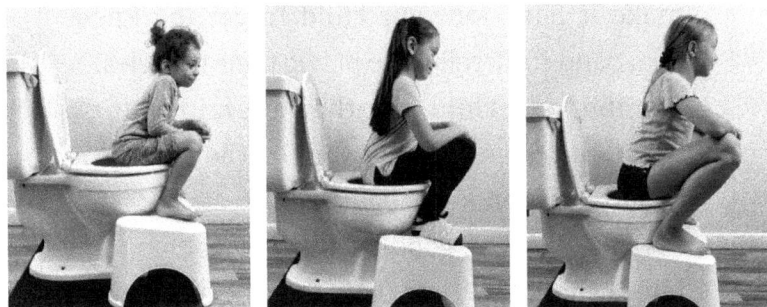

People are often shocked that I actually go into the bathroom with kids and their parents to teach them PPP on the actual toilet with their pants down. But here's the thing: I've learned that what a child does on the bench or on the toilet with pants on is very different from what they do with their pants down. Frequently, I'll teach a child during one session and ask them to go home to practice, but when I see them the following week they will have forgotten everything we talked about. Unless you work with your child and verify that they are actually in PPP on the toilet, it won't work.

Tips for successful PPP:

1. Teach your child to sit on the toilet first, then pull the stool forward from under the toilet to get it in place. Many kids try to pull the stool out and use it as a step to get onto the toilet. This leaves the stool too far in front of the toilet and will put your child's legs in the wrong position. It should only come an inch or two in front of the toilet.

2. Pants should come all the way down to the ankles. Pants that are still up around the knees

make it hard for your child to get the knees apart and fully relax the pelvic floor muscles.

3. Remind your child that they are mimicking a squat: they should sit forward on the toilet seat, just back far enough that their private parts are over the water. A good cue for kids is that their knees should be over their toes. I can't tell you how many kids report that they hate the Squatty Potty. When I ask these kids to show me how they're sitting, most are all the way back on the toilet with their knees up and their feet about a foot in front of their knees. They feel like they are going to fall into the toilet! They feel much more stable when they are forward on the seat.

4. Once you find the correct position for the feet on the stool, mark it. It is rare for kids to use the footprints on the Squatty Potty. These are meant for adults and are too wide for most kids.

It's important to note that I don't exactly know the optimal position for your child's low back for having a bowel movement. I have worked with hundreds of kids using biofeedback to assess the activity of the pelvic floor muscles. What we are looking for is a posture in which the muscles are stable and relaxed. For most kids, this is with their tailbone somewhat back, their pelvis tipped forward a bit, and the low back flat (not necessarily swayed like a cow … the cow pose is more useful teaching them to tip the pelvis forward and stick the tailbone back). A few of the kids I have worked with have been unable to relax their pelvic floor muscles in this posture, but they relax completely if I let them round their low back, or put their legs together, or bend forward and put their hands by their feet. Unfortunately, this posture isn't the most efficient for bearing down and fully emptying the rectum, so their poop might still get stuck despite the muscles relaxing.

Please try to help your child achieve the posture I have described above. If they tell you that they just can't poop in that position, but they can if they alter it a little bit, that's fine with me. You'll learn in the next chapter how to help them bear down, and they may find that, when using their belly correctly, they do better in perfect pooping posture.

CHAPTER 4 TAKEAWAYS:

- Human beings poop best when squatting. To make pooping as quick and pain-free as possible, it's best to come as close to squatting on the toilet as possible.
- "Perfect potty posture" takes practice! If you do not work with your child on this, they will likely end up in a posture that makes them less comfortable on the toilet.

CHAPTER 5

BEARING DOWN

W hen I first meet kids in the clinic, I ask them to show me what they do when they're having a bowel movement. The large majority of them have the same technique: they round their backs, suck in their tummies, and hold their breath. Already they are straining. The notion that they need to relax to have a better poop is totally foreign to them.

Many adults don't understand the need to relax, either. Many of us have struggled with constipation for so long that it seems totally normal to have to grunt and grimace while voiding. But it's not! A rectum that is functioning well actually has the ability to push out a soft, formed stool without a lot of help from the rest of the body. Of course, this is only true if the anal sphincter is also doing its job and relaxing while the rectum contracts. If your child has been struggling with constipation for a while, their rectum is likely stretched out and not as good at pushing stool out as it once was. The anal sphincter may have developed "dysynnergia," meaning it contracts to hold stool in when it should relax to let stool out.

For kids who are constipated, we need to teach them a new way of bearing down. It will involve using the upper abdominal muscles to help push and relaxing the muscles of the pelvic floor so they are no longer a barrier. Hopefully it will become second nature. When the rectum eventually shrinks down and starts effectively pushing out stool again, your child will be all set to have soft, easy poops with no straining.

To start, have your child lie on their back and put their hands on their belly. Tell them to breathe in through the nose and send the air all the way down to the belly, letting the air expand the belly like a balloon. Then ask them to breathe out through their mouth as if fogging up a mirror. As they breathe out, their belly should gradually shrink back down. Have them do it several times: inhale through the nose, inflate the belly like a balloon, exhale through the mouth, and gradually let the belly drift back down to normal size.

This is called diaphragmatic breathing or belly breathing. It helps:

1) Reduce the body's stress response. Many children have an undercurrent of stress in their lives and the body sometimes responds to stress by not pooping.

2) Draw the child's attention to the area of prime importance when re-learning how to feel poops—the belly.

3) Increase blood flow to the colon, which stimulates the colon to do its work of moving poop along.

4) Prepare kids for the work they are going to do on the toilet to push out poop.

Once your child knows how to belly breathe while lying on their back, transition them back to the bench they used to learn perfect pooping posture. Have them practice belly breathing in PPP. If they are sitting correctly, there should be a space between their thighs for their belly to expand into with each inhalation.

The next step is key: teach your child to practice "belly big, belly bigger." As they breathe in, they make their belly big. As they breathe out, with their foggy mirror breath, they need to make the belly even bigger. I'm not actually looking for their belly to get noticeably bigger when they exhale. When kids try to make their belly bigger when it's already been expanded by a belly breath, they actually make their belly hard. This firm belly means that the muscles we need to help push out a poop have become engaged.

To help kids who are struggling, I will get next to them and poke one finger into the side of their belly, midway between the belly button and their hip. Usually they will engage the correct muscles by trying to make their belly firm so I can't poke them. Another trick is to have your child say "haaaaard" while exhaling instead of doing a quiet foggy mirror breath. It's almost impossible to say a loud "haaaaa" sound without engaging your stomach muscles.

Side note: quite a few of my parents report that they now always know when their child is trying to poop because they will hear a loud "haaaaaard" coming from the bathroom. This brings me so much joy.

Pro tip: You should try this yourself before teaching your child. It is much easier to teach when you've felt it in your body.

It's super important that you don't linger too long practicing on the bench or on the toilet with the lid down. If they're doing this correctly, many kids will report that—lightbulb!—they need to poop! We don't want them to get that sensation and then have to stop everything, get all set up on the toilet, and then try again. So skip the bench all together, or just use it briefly and then move onto the toilet (with the lid up, pants down).

Getting the pelvic floor muscles on board:

I've mentioned that many kids have what's called pelvic floor muscle dyssynergia. This means that when the pelvic floor muscles should be relaxed (when a child is trying to pee or poop on the toilet), they actually contract to close the anus or urethra and hold in pee.

This condition can be super complicated to treat, requiring multiple PT sessions per week for weeks in a row. But here's what I've learned from my years of practice: for some kids with just chronic constipation (no daytime urinary incontinence, no history of urinary tract infections), re-teaching the pelvic floor muscles is often pretty easy.

First, you need to teach them what the pelvic floor muscles are. The pelvic floor muscles are a sling of muscles that surround your perineum—your private parts. These muscles do the important job of keeping everything that's in your stomach from falling down to the floor at your feet. They also work to hold pee and poop in when you're not on the toilet.

When your child is on the playground and gets an urge to pee or poop, their pelvic floor muscles contract, or shorten, and close around the urethra and anus—the holes the pee and poop come out of. Imagine your fingers pinching the end of a water balloon to keep the water from spraying out. When you get to the toilet, the muscles need to relax or loosen their hold on the urethra and anus so that pee and poop can come out. (I usually use "potty muscles" with younger kids, but I like to use the more anatomically correct terms—pelvic floor muscles, urethra, anus—with bigger kids. It reduces the giggle factor, and they usually appreciate the more scientific approach.)

To start teaching your child about the pelvic floor muscles, have them go back to belly breathing while lying on their back. Belly breathing can help kids learn to feel their pelvic floor muscles. As the child inhales, the pelvic floor should descend, and when they exhale, the pelvic floor muscles should rise back up. This may not be the case for your child – sometimes the pelvic floor is tight and doesn't move in this way – but it's worth asking them to pay attention to their bottom and see if they can feel any movement of the muscles while breathing.

Next, ask them to use their potty muscles to close the hole that the poop comes out of. Usually, when first asked to do this, they will tighten their butt muscles and legs and even arch their back a little. They will often hold their breath, too. They shouldn't do any of this! Here are the cues that work best for me when asking kids to contract their pelvic floor muscles:

- Pull up and close the hole the poop comes out of.
- Think of pulling all of your private parts up into your belly.

- Pretend there's a fart that wants to come out, but you don't want to let it out and you can't move because you're playing the statue game.

I do NOT recommend using the verbs "squeeze," or "tighten." These words just seem to get kids to contract every muscle in their body to help.

Practice these exercises with you sitting on the edge of a bed and your child laying down with their legs over your lap. Your legs will feel when your child's legs contract to help the pelvic floor muscles along. You can also put one hand on your child's belly to feel when they are using their abdominal muscles or holding their breath to help. Tell your child to keep their entire body quiet or still and to just use the tiny muscles between the legs to pull up and close the anus. With younger kids, I will laugh when I feel their legs twitch and say "Oh! Your legs are so helpful today! But no thanks, legs, it's just the potty muscles that need to work today."

Here's the thing: if they are doing this correctly, you won't be able to tell. I've found that most of my kids with chronic constipation are pretty easy to teach. You just have to find the right words and make sure they know what you're asking them to do. If they are struggling, find a physical therapist who will be able to teach them this skill.

Once your child feels as though they understand how to contract and relax the pelvic floor muscles, they should practice this skill for a few days in a row, lying on their back with their legs over your lap. Have them do ten quick con-tractions (pull up, then relax quickly) in a row, then have them do a few longer (5-10 second) contractions. If they find it pretty easy when they're lying down, have them do it sitting up. Car rides are a great place to practice this.

After a few days of practice, it's time for them to bring this awareness of the pelvic floor muscles to the toilet when they're having a bowel movement. I like to have kids sit on the toilet in perfect pooping posture, then do 5-10 quick contractions before they start trying to bear down. While I wouldn't advocate for a lot of practicing of pelvic floor muscles on the toilet (and I would never ask a child to practice these contractions by stopping the flow of urine), I believe a few quick contractions are very useful. It's really important that kids take a second to feel what is happening on their bottom when their potty muscles contract and relax: they pull up and the anus closes, they relax and the anus comes down and opens up a little.

When you child indicates that they understand the pulling up to contract and the letting down to relax, they then need to feel what the anus is doing when they are bearing down. Ask them to exhale, keep their belly big and hard, and bear down. They should feel their pelvic floor muscles staying low and relaxed when they are trying to push poop out. If they feel their potty muscles contract and their anus pull up into their body while they are trying to poop, then they need more practice relaxing.

Putting it all together:

So here is what should happen every time your child sits to try to have a bowel movement:

1) They get into perfect pooping posture.
2) They do a few quick contractions of the pelvic floor muscles to remind their brain what it feels like to

relax the pelvic floor muscles, let the anus descend, and open so a poop can come out.

3) They breathe in and make their belly big.

4) They breathe out, make their belly bigger and harder, relax the pelvic floor muscles, and try to push out a poop. They should not hold their breath while doing this! With the foggy mirror breath exhale or by saying "haaaaard," they should be breathing long and slow.

5) They do this a few times in a row, then they stay in PPP but take a little break from all the belly breathing. After a bit, they do 3-5 more breaths in a row.

What is biofeedback?

Physical therapists use biofeedback to teach kids about the pelvic floor muscles. This involves putting gel electrodes (I tell the kids they are stickers) on the skin of their bottoms on either side of the anus. Some therapists will also use a sticker on the abdominal muscles to teach kids to coordinate the belly and the bottom when trying to poop. The electrodes are then hooked up to a computer, and the child can watch on the screen as they contract and relax these muscles.

Biofeedback is a wonderful tool! I can use all sorts of words to try to teach kids about their pelvic floor muscles, but biofeedback gives them instant visual feedback when they use these muscles. Kids learn quickly and painlessly how to use these muscles appropriately.

Most common questions from kids about biofeedback:

1) Will it hurt? Well, no and yes. No, the electrodes don't hurt and doing the biofeedback is entirely painless. But ... yes, taking the stickers off your bottom might hurt a little. Less than taking off a bandage, but a little.

2) Will it shock me? No. The stickers only "read" your muscle activity; they don't send any energy into your body.

3) Will it be embarrassing? Only for a minute. Once the stickers are where they are supposed to be, usually the therapist will have you pull your clothes back up and you'll be fully dressed while you're learning.

Most kids are embarrassed the first time they get biofeedback, but then they get used to it. They learn that it's helping, so they're not embarrassed for long. Also, the PT will explain that PTs are a type of doctor, and the only people who ever get to look at your child's bottom are doctors and their parents or caregivers.

Research show that using biofeedback with kids is highly effective to treat urinary incontinence. With chronic constipation, the evidence is less conclusive. I believe that's because chronic constipation almost always involves more than just pelvic floor dysfunction. Just as laxatives alone won't cure constipation, neither will biofeedback alone.

CHAPTER 5 TAKEAWAYS

- Once a child has learned how to sit in "perfect potty posture", they need to learn to use their belly muscles to push out poop while keeping their pelvic floor muscles relaxed.

- Teaching your child to do a pelvic floor muscle contraction is helpful because they will learn what it feels like to use the pelvic floor muscles to hold in pee or poop, and then to relax them while bearing down.

- Changing your child's technique for bearing down will take some practice. It will also take time and focus. If they struggle with this technique, find a physical therapist who uses biofeedback to teach kids to use the pelvic floor muscles.

CHAPTER 6

HOW TO MOVE

I said earlier that diet and exercise alone can't fix constipation, but it's still important to pay attention to these areas. This chapter will focus on specific exercises your child can do to set them up for quicker, easier bowel movements.

This is my go-to list of exercises to help kids poop better. They are easy to explain, quick to execute, and frequently very effective at producing at least one bowel movement per day. If possible, kids should do these exercises between eating and sitting to try to have a bowel movement. If it's not possible to do after a meal, do them anytime and just have your kid sit on the toilet after exercising.

To simplify things, I've grouped the exercises into three categories: aerobic, strengthening, and then stretch/relax. Your child should pick two from each category.

Aerobic:
- Jumping jacks: do 30 at a normal pace, rest for 20 seconds, then do 15 at a record-setting pace. Rest for

another 20 seconds, then do another 15 at a record-setting pace.

- Jumping sideways up and down from the bottom stair: do 10 jumps facing one direction, then 10 jumps facing the other direction. Rest for 30 seconds, then do 10 more jumps each way.

- Running outdoors: Pick a safe, close to home route to jog (i.e. front door to end of driveway over and over again, front door to corner of the block and back). Jog for one continuous minute and then rest a minute. Then do some sprints: run super fast for 15 seconds, rest for 30 seconds. Repeat this three times in a row. (Instead of time, you could use distances: run to the end of the driveway and back twice, then rest.) End with another slow jog for a minute.

- High knees running in place: Normal pace for 30 seconds, rest; fast pace for 15 seconds with 30 seconds rest in between, three times. Then normal pace for another 30 seconds.

- Frog jumps: squat all the way to the floor like a frog (heels on the ground if you can). Jump up and reach up to touch the ceiling, then come back down to the frog squat. Do ten in a row. You can move forward down the hallway or just do them in place. Bonus for saying "ribbit" with each jump!

Strengthening:

- Bicycles: Lie on your back, hands behind head, knees bent with feet off the floor. Bring your right elbow to the left knee while the right leg goes straight (but doesn't touch the floor). Then switch legs and bring the left elbow to the right knee. Do ten in a row, then rest, then do another set of 10.

- *This can be hard for beginners (and those low-tone kids I mentioned earlier). If your child is struggling, they can keep their feet on the floor and just lift one knee at a time to the opposite elbow.*

- Planks: A plank is when you put all of your weight on your toes and your forearms and keep the rest of your body as straight and strong as a board. This means the head, shoulders, bottom and heels should make a straight, tilted line. Hold a plank for 10 seconds, rest, then do it again. As they get better, your child should be able to hold a plank for 20-30 seconds at a time— but only if they aren't swaying their back!

  - *The hardest part about planks for the kids I work with is keeping their backs from swaying like a cow's back. Cue your kid to make sure their core is super strong by tapping on the sides of their belly to see if their core muscles are engaged. Also, put your hand over their low back and tell them to press their low back (not their bottom!) up into your hand. When you do this, you can tell them to do a little tail tuck like they did when making a camel's hump to learn PPP.*

  - *If your child is struggling with plank, have them do it on their knees. Or, they can do a "bear plank," in which they start on their hands and knees with a flat back (like for camel/cow) and then just tuck their toes and lift their knees. Hold for 10 seconds. It's important that your child feels their belly muscles working during this exercise.*

- Popcorn: Lie on your back and curl up into a popcorn seed: lift your head and hug your knees to your chest with both arms. Then "pop," bringing your arms and your legs out to the side so you're an expanded version of yourself, but don't lower your head and don't let your arms and legs go all the way down to the ground. Hold the popped position, then curl back up into a seed. Do 10 pops in a row if you can.
- Bird-dogs: Get on your hands and knees with a flat back. Keeping your back flat and level the whole time, slowly point your left hand forward. Then, slowly kick your right leg back. Don't let your low back sway! You should feel your belly muscles working. Hold for five seconds, then come back to hands and knees. Then switch to the other side. Do five on each side, for five seconds each.
  - *The biggest pitfalls in this exercise are letting the low back sway or letting the hip drop. I always put my hands on their hips to remind them to keep the hips level. You should do this too. Once they get stronger, they won't need your hands to help them.*
  - *Put a book or a plastic plate on their back so they remember not to "tip the table."*
  - *If keeping the back strong and level is too hard, just do this exercise with the legs to begin with. Add the arms as they get stronger.*
- Wide-legged squats: stand with your feet a little bit wider than your hips, feet pointing out a little bit. Put your arms straight in front of you or put your hands on your hips. Slowly squat down so your bottom is about a foot from the ground. Then slowly come back

up. Try to do as many of these as you can, until your legs feel like they couldn't manage another squat even if someone gave them $10.

Stretch/relax

- Static frog squat: Squat like a frog, with your heels on the floor. Read a book, do a puzzle, or draw on a tablet for 2 minutes.
  - *Keeping their heels on the floor can be super hard for some kids! If this is the case for your child, ask them to stand, bend their knees slightly, reach down and touch the floor with their hands, and then lower their bottom. Sometimes this helps keep them from popping up onto their toes. You can also put a pencil across the front of their ankle and ask them to use their shin muscles to try to squish the pencil between their shin and the top of their foot.*
  - *Sometimes a child's calf muscles are simply too tight to keep the heels on the floor. If this is the case, roll up a towel and have them stand with their heels on the towel, forefeet on the floor. Then come down into a squat as described above.*
- Child's pose: Sit on your heels with your knees and feet a little wider apart than your hips. Lean forward and put your head on the floor in front of your knees. Your arms can go at your sides or straight in front of you. Breathe deeply and send all that fresh air way down to your low back. Stay in this position for 1-2 minutes.
- Happy baby pose: Lie on your back and raise your bent knees up in the air like a baby getting its diaper

changed. Grab your feet and pull your bent knees down and out to the side. Keep your head on the ground and just relax into this stretch for a minute or so.

- Figure four stretch: Lie on your back with your knees bent, feet on the floor. Cross your left ankle over your right knee. Then grab your right thigh with both hands (you'll put your left hand between your legs and your right hand around the outside of your right leg) and pull your thigh up towards your chest. You don't have to get all the way to your chest, just until you feel a stretch on the outside of your left hip. Hold for about one minute on the one side, then switch legs and stretch the same way, but this time with your right ankle on your left knee.

- Camel/cow: Start on your hands and knees with a flat back. Breathe in and arch your back like you're making a camel's hump. Hold for a second or two, then breathe out and sway your back like a cow's belly. Do this slowly and with focus for 10 breaths. Then switch and do the opposite: breathe in and sway your back like a cow, then breathe out and arch your back like a camel.

  ○ *Usually in yoga the instructor will ask you to inhale for cow and exhale for camel. This is fine, but I also like to switch it up and inhale while making the camel's hump. It gives a little bit of an extra stretch to the mid-back.*

  ○ *Typically in yoga these poses are called cat and cow. I've always said "camel" to my patients because, to me, making a camel's hump is easy to visualize. So I'm sticking with it, but you can certainly use "cat" if that's what you are used to.*

- Belly breathing on your back: Lie on your back, hands on your belly, eyes closed. Breathe in through your nose like you're smelling flowers and feel your belly expand with the air you just inhaled. Breathe out through your mouth like you're fogging up a mirror or blowing out a candle. Let your belly float back down to where it started.

  o *If you child finds belly breathing to be easy, challenge them to breathe in for four seconds, hold for four seconds, and breathe out for eight seconds. This is an excellent way to calm down the body and the mind.*

Remember: Have your child do these exercises at least once a day, preferably after a meal. After doing them, have your child sit on the toilet in perfect pooping posture. If they find that they always have a BM at a certain time of day, have them do these exercises right at that time (for example, if they always poop after school, make it their routine that they do these exercises as soon as they get home from school before they sit).

Also, try to make sure they aren't doing the same exercises every day. Mixing it up will keep things interesting, and they might find that one exercise in particular helps them have better poops.

One final thing: try to make a small amount of moderate exercise a part of your family's daily life. Take walks, go to the park and shoot baskets or hit tennis balls, do an on-line strengthening class. Share with your children that you're all going to try to do some exercise every day, because everybody needs exercise (not just your kid with constipation issues). Exercise helps you learn, helps your mood, helps your heart and lungs stay strong ... see if you can use your child's struggles with constipation to help everyone in your family get healthier. It will be a constipation silver lining!

CHAPTER 6 TAKEAWAYS:

- While exercise alone won't cure constipation, certain exercises can set your child up for easier, more frequent bowel movements.
- Your child should choose an aerobic activity, a strengthening activity and a stretching activity to do between eating a meal and sitting to try to poop.
- The exercises in this chapter promote colonic motility, relax the pelvic floor muscles, and make sitting in Perfect Potty Posture easier. They are like pressing a "turbo boost" button on your child's recovery from chronic constipation.

CHAPTER 7

RECOGNIZING AND MANAGING STRESS

Overfilled classrooms, social media, busy parents, a different extracurricular activity every day after school. Kids have so much to manage already. And *your* kid has the added bonus of having "constipation stress" on top of everything else.

It's a thing! Once a kid has noted a challenge with pooping—it hurts, it causes stomach aches, it takes too much time, it's embarrassing—they can easily start having constipation stress. And, like all other stressors in life, constipation stress can cause ... you guessed it: constipation! So in addition to the constipation cycle we've already described (backup of stool stretching out the rectum and colon, causing an even greater backup of stool), there's a constipation stress cycle we need to break as well.

Defining stress

Keep it simple for your kids: Stress is what they feel when they are scared, worried, or overloaded. Everybody feels stress, kids and adults. Having some stress is good for us: if you are stressed out about a test, you might study a little harder and get a better grade than you would have if you hadn't stressed a bit. Too much stress is not good for us: If you are so stressed out about the test that you can't sleep, you might do worse than you would have.

I like to teach kids about stress by describing my "stress bucket." (This concept is courtesy of my allergy doctor, who similarly described a person's "allergy bucket.") I have a stress bucket that I carry around with me. All of the stressors in my life go into it: When my kids are sluggish and can't get ready for school on time and we're all late, that goes into my stress bucket. When my dad gets sick and I need to go to the doctor with him, another stress goes into the bucket. When we have a bill to pay that we weren't expecting, more stress fills the bucket. I can handle my stress bucket pretty well—until it overflows.

When I have too much stress and my stress bucket overflows, my body starts showing signs of stress. For me, I get a gurgly stomach, I miss the urge to have my morning bowel movement, I take shallow breaths and am likely to feel tired. My actions show the stress as well: I have a shorter fuse and tend to snap at my family members more than I'd like. I also bite my nails.

Many kids have one or a few of the following physical and behavioral symptoms when their stress buckets are full:

- Stomachaches
- Headaches
- Sweaty palms

- Difficulty falling asleep or staying asleep
- Wanting to eat too much or not wanting to eat at all
- Hyperactivity
- Behaviors such as yelling, kicking or punching

Your kid might display some of these symptoms or none at all. It's important to talk with them to help them identify stress and their response to it.

I'd like you to do an activity with your kid (or your whole family, as this doesn't just apply to constipated kids). First, everybody makes a list of all the things that fill their stress buckets. Then, everybody makes a list of all the ways their bodies react when their stress buckets overflow. Share your lists with your kids and have them share with you. Remember, this isn't about you trying to fix things for your kid; it's just about helping everybody get to know more about everybody else's bucket. Constipation aside, it's nice to know these things about the people you live with!

If your child can't come up with any of the ways their bodies respond to stress, you might suggest some of the common responses that I listed above. You also might point out that they have chronic constipation, and that's strongly linked to stress. This can be an ongoing conversation you have with them over the next few months as you treat the constipation.

Managing stress:

Now that your child has a better understanding of what stress is and how they respond to it, it's time to develop strategies for managing the stress. First, how can you manage stressful situations in the moment? Second, what changes can you make in life to reduce the overall stress level?

What to do in the moment?

DEEP BREATHING: Stressful situations result in a spike in the hormone cortisol in the body. Cortisol is a "flight or fight" hormone, and too much of it can be damaging. Deep breathing, like what we already practiced in Chapter 5, will reduce the cortisol flowing through your body. The best thing is, you can practice deep breathing anywhere. When your classroom is getting crazy and you can feel yourself getting tense, take some deep belly breaths. When your family is in the car and everybody is talking at once, breathe deeply. Once you have belly breathing down, try to exhale slightly longer than you inhale (breathe in for four seconds and out for six seconds, for example). Be sure to breathe in through the nose (if possible) and out through the mouth.

EXERCISE: Go for a hike, jog or run. Do a bunch of jumping jacks. Do a kids yoga video online. Have a family dance party. Second to deep breathing, exercise is probably the surest way to reduce the effect of stress on the body.

WRITE: Find a piece of paper and pencil, sit down at the table, and write. It doesn't matter what you write about. You can write a journal, a story, or just whatever thoughts come to mind. You can crumple it up into a ball and toss it when you're done if you want. If something is bothering you, trying writing a story about a character who feels the way you do.

ART: This can be anything, as long as it doesn't make you feel bad for not being an artist or provide more stress about how creative you are. Find a photo of a person you love and try to sketch their face. Make a slideshow of your favorite photos on the computer. Compose a song on your recorder.

ZONE OUT: Massage a stress ball. Play Tetris or some other mindless game. Color in a coloring book. Set a timer and do something mindless for 15 minutes and see how it makes you feel.

How to lower overall stress levels

It might be that your child is just particularly susceptible to stress. Or it might be that their life really is super stressful. Either way, your family might have to make some changes to help reduce your child's stress levels.

Make sure everybody is getting enough sleep: Sleep deprivation is a thing, and, to go back to the bucket analogy, not enough sleep makes your stress bucket smaller. Kids shouldn't have any electronics one hour before bedtime. They should have a regular bedtime, and it should be early enough that they can wake up early enough to have a morning routine that includes sitting on the toilet before school.

Think about limiting activities: As you likely know, it doesn't take too many activities to feel like your family is constantly running from place to place. In our family, we limited extracurriculars to one musical instrument and one sport, and that felt manageable, but then there was theater camp and then there was an after-school imagination club and then there was a school running club. Before we knew it, we were running around constantly and had no time to cook, eat together, play games or go for family walks. It's hard to say no to your kids when they want to do something that's good for them but finding time to relax together every single day is also healthy and good for them.

See what can be changed at school. If your child indicates that their classroom is stressful, they likely aren't the only kid in the class who feels that way. Talk with the teacher to see if they can implement a few stress-relieving activities into the day: deep breathing, stretching breaks, mindfulness minutes. Teachers have so many ideas on how to de-stress a classroom; sometimes they might just need to be made aware that your child is struggling.

It might be helpful for your entire family to do a guided relaxation exercise once a week. There are many guided relaxation videos available on the Web, and several apps that have audio-only relaxation scripts. In addition to lowering overall stress, these exercises might help your child learn the differences in how their body feels from one day to the next. Identifying the changes, and figuring out what led to them are huge steps in regaining urge awareness for bowel movements.

It's important to note that many of the ways to reduce your child's stress levels are going to involve you changing your life in a few ways. Through my own parenting, I've come to believe that kids' stress levels are directly proportional to parental stress levels. I don't say that to judge, just to acknowledge what I believe to be a reality for many families. Make a few, small, family-wide changes. You'll know you're on the right track if things get slightly better.

How to lower constipation stress:

Constipation stress is tough: Not only is there the physical stress of not having regular bowel movements, but often there is an overwhelming feeling of blame and guilt and failure that magnify all the other stressors. This situation gets worse if fecal incontinence is involved.

The first thing to do is to practice forgiveness with everyone involved: nobody is to blame, nobody knew what to do, and nobody can manage all the elements of constipation (diet, exercise, medicines, schedule) perfectly. So be kind to each other, expect some slip-ups and regressions, and try your best.

The second thing is to reassure your child that you will work with your doctor to ensure that your child will never have a poop that hurts again. Or not one that hurts seriously. Your child needs to be able to relax to have a bowel movement, and they won't relax unless they are sure it is safe to do so.

Then you have to address all of the other likely constipation stressors: is the bathroom at school sometimes dirty? Are the other students all going through a phase in which they laugh when someone has to poop? Is the light too bright in the bathroom? Is there too much going on in the rest of the house when your child is sitting to poop, and are they distracted?

I once had a patient tell me that she was about to poop, but then she saw a bug creeping across the bathroom floor and her poop stopped coming out. She wasn't scared—it was just too distracting to watch that bug and poop at the same time. You won't know what your child is feeling until you ask. And you won't know what to do about it until you brainstorm with your child. Maybe they need noise-cancelling headphones in the bathroom. Maybe they need classical music. Maybe the rest of the family needs to go outside (eventually your child will have to be able to poop with other people in the house, but we're talking baby steps right now).

Some kids just need everybody to stop talking about their poop! This can be hard, because it's the rare child that can handle everything related to their constipation management on their own. But it's important to respect this feeling in your child. I'm a huge fan of vibrating watches that will remind your child to use the restroom on a schedule. Your child's body isn't giving them the signals they need to poop, and your child is tired of your constant reminders to sit. The watch replaces both of those signals and gives your child a break from the nagging.

If your child is old enough, you can give them some autonomy over their chart. Tape it on the inside of a bathroom cabinet door and tell them that you are just going to check it once a day to make sure they did everything (they still need you as a coach, after all). Ask your child what they would like to be reminded about and what they want to try to accomplish all on their own. Have weekly meetings to see how things are working out and what needs to be changed.

Side note on anxiety

We need to differentiate between stress and anxiety. Stress is a natural response to a challenge: your kid really wants to poop, and they can't. They don't feel good, and that stresses them out. Or they are being challenged in new ways at school; it's not easy and they are stressed about it.

Anxiety is a persistent fear of the unknown, even when there is no immediate threat or challenge. An anxious child might think constantly about a meteor hitting their house. There is no immediate threat of a meteor, and the likelihood is low, but the child plans for it as though it is inevitable. Another child also might have a disproportionately long and intense response to challenging situations: screaming for hours before entering their kindergarten classroom for the first time or agonizing for days over what to bring to an upcoming birthday party.

I mentioned earlier a certain subset of my patients that are "parent pleasers." These kids want to do everything right. Their teachers love them, they get good grades and excel in lots of areas. When you meet them, they do not seem stressed out, but they can struggle with constipation (and often urinary incontinence as well). I've come to realize that "parent pleaser" kids often have underlying, mostly invisible anxiety. It's not the anxiety we typically think of, but it's real, and their bowel and bladder issues improve once the anxiety is addressed.

Chronic, persistent anxiety can be treated. Some signs that your child might need help include being worried more often than not and being worried about events that don't typically cause much stress in kids: a play date, recess, current events, etc. If you feel your child might be struggling with real anxiety, getting them to a mental health therapist is a gift you can give that will last their entire life.

CHAPTER 7 TAKEAWAYS

- Stress causes physiological changes that often make constipation worse.
- You and your child should work together to identify causes of stress in your child's life.
- Your child needs tools to deal with stress, both in-the-moment and in the long-term.
- If you feel your child's stress may be indicative of an underlying anxiety problem, seek help from a mental health professional.

CHAPTER 8

HOW TO EAT

P oop comes from the food you eat, so what your child eats does make a difference in their constipation. While I strongly believe that medications are necessary for managing constipation, improving diet is key in preventing regression and successfully weaning a child off laxatives.

You will find all sorts of advice online on how to eat better for constipation, but a lot of it is not anchored in research. Instead of giving you a specific list of foods to eat and another one of foods not to eat, I'd like you to try to follow some broad food rules:

1) Snacks should mostly be fruit, veggies, or nuts, accompanied by a glass of water.

2) Meals should follow the USDA "choose your plate" guidelines: ¼ of the plate should be fruit, ¼ of the plate veggies, ¼ protein, and ¼ grain.

3) Buy whole wheat or whole grain pasta, bread and tortillas, and use brown rice instead of white.

4) Do not keep highly processed snack foods in the house. By this, I mean, goldfish crackers, sandwich cookies, gummy snacks, sweet cereals, potato chips, etc.

5) Encourage your child to slow down between bites and to chew food well.

6) Always drink a glass of water with meals and with snacks.

I know that this is a lot to take in. No household is going to be able to follow all of these rules all at the same time. But consider the logic behind each rule and see if you can't try to follow one or two for now and a few more down the road.

Rule #1: Snack time is the hardest time to prevent kids from eating junk. If they have strict guidelines that they can only snack on fruit and veggies, they will find it is much easier to get close to that goal of 7 servings of fruits and veggies a day. Conversely, if they are allowed to snack on chips and crackers, that goal might seem impossible. Another benefit to snacking only on produce and nuts is that your child just might end up snacking less. This is a good thing—remember, we are trying to trigger that gastrocolic reflex by letting the stomach shrink and then expand with a full meal. Less snacking overall gives that reflex more of a chance to work.

Rule #2: The Choose My Plate guidelines from the USDA's Center for Nutrition Policy and Promotion give kids and parents a super-simple graphic on which to model their meals.

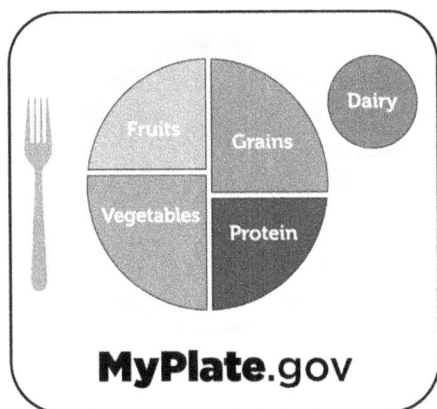

MyPlate.gov

You can study the plate or you can just follow this guideline: half of *every* meal should be fruit and vegetables. Americans, kids included, do not eat enough fiber. As a general rule, your child should eat her age plus five in grams of fiber per day. The easiest way to accomplish this lofty goal is to increase the number of fruits and veggies they eat.

Kids (and their parents) are often shocked when I say that the Choose My Plate guidelines apply to breakfast as well! For years my daughter ate a couple of carrot sticks with her breakfast. (She would still, except that she is too old now for me to control that part of her life.) I knew that she struggled with getting enough fruit and vegetables. I knew the snacks served in her grade school classrooms were junk that she was thrilled to devour, and I knew that she had to take every opportunity to eat roughage.

Side note on the USDA guidelines

I'm not thrilled about the suggestion that every meal should be accompanied by a glass of milk. But I love the idea that we should all be drinking *something* with every meal. My preference is water, but unsweetened almond, soy or oat milk are also good choices.

Rule #3: Switching to whole grains is the other way to get to adequate fiber consumption. If you haven't recently tried alternative pastas, breads and tortillas that are made with whole wheat or whole grain flours, you should! I remember the days when these variations were dry and crumbly and completely unsuitable as a substitute for white flour products. This is not the case anymore. Barilla makes a whole grain pasta that also has pea protein (a fiber and protein bonus!) that can pass for regular pasta with most kids. Brown rice takes some getting used to, but in my family we are at the point where we much prefer brown rice (and other grains, such as farro and barley) to white rice.

Ask your kid to go on a tasting adventure with you and see if you can find products that they can tolerate. Remind them: they are trying to eat a little different so they can feel better overall. These different foods might take an adjustment, but if your child has an open mind and knows why the change matters, they might be more open to it.

Rule #4:   Of all of these rules, the fourth one may be the most important and the hardest to follow. You have to remove the temptation! As adults, we may be able to handle having an open bag of potato chips in the cupboard and not scarfing it down in the five minutes after we get home from work. (I can't, but maybe you can.) But kids just don't have that executive function yet. If they are home without supervision, they are going to eat the most tempting, snackable foods in the house. If you have chips, they will find the chips. If you have chocolate, they will find the chocolate.

   Note: You are likely to see an increase in poor behavior when you make this change. Your child is going to feel like you do when you go to a vending machine, put in your money, and the bag of candy gets stuck: they may scream, punch the pantry door, and shake you down for a sweet or salty snack. Don't give in! Remind them (and yourself) that they don't likely *need* a snack to survive, and, if they do, there are apples in the fridge. After a while, your family will get used to this new reality.

Rule #5:   The process of digestion—breaking down food into nutrients and waste (poop)—starts in the mouth. Many kids, and especially picky eaters, have a tendency to stuff food into their mouth, chew it minimally, and swallow big lumpy balls of food. Once food gets into the stomach, it mixes with stomach acids to make a runny soup. If your child doesn't chew their food, the soup is more like a stew, and the body has to work harder to break down larger lumps of unchewed food. Those lumps, especially if they consist of processed white flour, can block up the digestive track even more. Chewing food thoroughly, and swallowing smaller amounts, will set the rest of the digestive track up for success.

Rule #6: Drinking enough water is essential to keeping stool soft. If your body is dehydrated, your super-smart sense of homeostasis is going to tell your body to conserve water wherever it can be found. Guess what holds a lot of water? Stool going through the large intestine. So one of the first things that happens when we become dehydrated is that our body pulls water from the large intestine, turning our poop into hard, dried out turds.

I often work with kids who tell me that they drink tons of water. Their parents elaborate: she gets home after school and just chugs a 24-ounce water bottle! In my follow-up questions, I learn that she doesn't usually drink *any* water between waking up and getting home from school. Unfortunately, drinking 24 ounces in one gulp is not an effective way to prevent dehydrated BMs. Your body needs a little bit of water all day long, because your heart is beating and your muscles are working all day long. Depending on the weather and your child's activity level, they can become dehydrated quickly. It took me years as a therapist to realize that one of the reasons my kids were regressing during our hot summer months was likely that they were outside playing for hours at a time without rehydrating.

Some kids naturally drink lots of water all day long, and some need constant reminders. I can't fully explain why this is, but I think it's because some kids are better at noticing how their body feels. Kids with chronic constipation often have trouble noticing their body signals, thirst included. We need to give them strategies. A rule that they drink a full glass (8-12 ounces) of water with every meal is a good place to start. Another rule should be that they carry a 16-ounce water bottle to school and that they drink it all by the end of the day. Remember to explain the reasoning behind these rules: drinking smaller amounts of water all day long will help them feel better.

Side notes on diet

Picky eating: I hope you do not have a child who is a very picky eater. Given that you have a child with chronic constipation, though, the odds are fairly good that you do. I have a very picky eater and making sure her diet is well-balanced takes up a surprisingly large amount of our parenting brain space.

You're certainly not going to be able to force your picky eater to eat certain foods. But you might be able to entice her by starting with what she does like. If she only eats grapes, maybe you can find another round fruit for her to try (blueberries?

cherry tomatoes?). If she only eats baby carrots, maybe she'll try an orange bell pepper that has been cut to the same size and shape. Does she like apples? Maybe she'll like another super crunchy food like a carrot. This is called Food Chaining, and pediatric occupational therapists have loads of tricks to help your child take one small adventurous food step after another. I'll talk more about occupational therapists in Chapter 9.

A final note on picky eating: try to cut out as many liquid calories as possible, especially milk. Many picky eaters will drink 4-5 glasses of milk a day. Not only is milk constipating (see below), but it also fills your child up. If a child is allowed endless amounts of milk, they will not be hungry for the whole grains, fruits, and vegetables they need.

Cow's Milk: It is well-established that cow's milk causes or contributes to constipation in humans. Many of the parents I work with report that the constipation started when the child started drinking cow's milk. But once that initial constipation is resolved (or *seems to be resolved*, as we've discussed that new stool can move around old stool and make a child seem less constipated), the child continues to drink cow's milk and eat cheese.

If your child is still struggling with having a regular bowel movement after you have done a cleanout and implemented a daily laxative routine, try cutting out dairy. It's not easy, but it is a fairly straightforward intervention. Cut out *all* dairy for three or four weeks. You might not notice an immediate difference, but you may over time. Or you may only notice that eliminating dairy made a difference when you add it back into the diet after eliminating it, and your child suddenly isn't pooping as well.

Fiber additives: There is not a lot of research regarding the use of fiber supplements in the pediatric population. In my experience, physicians are not likely to recommend adding a bulk-forming fiber in kids. This could be because a stretched-out colon just doesn't have the push power (the motility) to move a bolus of rough fiber through the system. It could also be that the supplements only work if a person also drinks sufficient water, which many constipated kids don't do. Finally, a bulk-forming fiber could easily get stuck behind a ball of stool in the rectum, making the back-up even worse.

I usually advise my patients to hold off on fiber supplements until they are fairly certain they are cleaned out. Remember, this can take several months of regular clean-outs and laxative use. Once they want to try cutting back on the laxatives, the research in adults suggests that psyllium seed husks is the most effective fiber supplement. Psyllium has a good balance of soluble and insoluble fiber, which means it softens the poop and pushes it through the system. When giving it to kids, keep the following guidelines in mind:

- Start with a small amount, like ½ to 1 tsp per day. Starting with too large an addition of fiber can lead to worsened constipation, cramping, bloating and gas.

- Always drink fiber supplements with plenty of water and continue to drink water regularly throughout the day.
- Take supplements at the same time of day, if possible. Do it for two weeks in a row, at least, so the body can adapt to the additional fiber.

On fiber gummies: Most fiber gummies contain soluble fiber, which means it forms a gel and holds water in your digestive system. They do not have insoluble fiber, which is helpful in pushing stool through the system. Psyllium is generally considered to be a more effective fiber supplement. But you may have a child who won't eat psyllium, so the gummies are an attractive alternative.

Often the fiber in gummies comes from inulin or other types of sugars. I have certainly had patients who swear by fiber gummies for maintaining regularity. But you should know that these types of sugars sometimes cause gas and stomach aches. And because of the large variety of soluble fibers used to make them, you may find one brand that works very well while another seems to have no effect. Follow the above suggestions for psyllium when adding fiber gummies to your child's regimen.

What about probiotics?

Probiotics are the good bacteria and yeasts that live in your body and help it function. You have probably seen probiotic supplements in the grocery store. Most of the research on probiotics has shown that they can be effective at treating diarrhea. Whether or not they are effective in treating constipation is less clear. One study shows that *bifidobacterium lactis* is effective at increasing the frequency of bowel movements. Other studies say that *L. rhamnosus* does the job. This research is promising, but a lot more needs to be done. A systematic review of the literature published in 2020 concluded that there just isn't enough evidence to support one probiotic recommendation for constipation.

Probiotics are also generally expensive, and they vary greatly in the types and concentration of bacteria they contain. On the whole, I encourage families to try probiotics if they are willing to give a consistent dose for a few weeks and if they are economically able. It's important to remember a few things:

- Utilize a name brand that has a reputation for quality. Cultivating and transporting live and active probiotic strains is a highly technical process. Inexpensive or store brands may not have gone through a rigorous quality control check.
- Look for products that have at least one billion CFU (colony-forming units) per dose.
- Try a probiotic for a few weeks before making a decision about its effectiveness. It usually takes at least a couple of weeks to see results.
- Do some research to make sure you are choosing a strain that is intended to help with constipation. Many out there have been found to help with diarrhea.
- Tell your doctor that your child is taking probiotics. Do not give your kid probiotics if they have a compromised immune system or Crohn's disease.

If you find a probiotic that seems to work for your child, great! If you don't see a difference after a few weeks, switch to a different brand or just skip probiotics for now. They might be more effective later as the constipation becomes less severe.

You should also consider giving your child more food with naturally occurring probiotics. These include yogurt (but not yogurt with thickeners like gelatin in it, this can be constipating and usually means the yogurt has less live and active cultures in it), sauerkraut, kimchi, kefir, and kombucha.

While we're talking probiotics, we should discuss "prebiotic" foods as well. Prebiotic foods contain fiber that the body can't digest. This fiber's job is to feed the bacteria that exist in the gut. The study of prebiotics is in its infancy, but more and more researchers are finding that consuming prebiotic foods is essential for maintaining the right balance of bacteria in the gut. Prebiotic foods include whole grains, onions, garlic, artichokes, leafy greens and asparagus. It's worth trying to add some of these foods to your child's diet in addition to the probiotic supplements.

In closing up this chapter on food, I'd like to make one thing clear: your child's *chronic* constipation was not caused by diet alone, and you won't be able to cure it by changing only their diet. So try your best to improve what your child eats, but don't think that you've lost all progress when she has cake, fries and hot dogs all weekend long at her grandparents' house.

CHAPTER 8 TAKEAWAYS

- Use the USDA Choose My Plate campaign as a guide for every meal.
- Make gradual changes in your family's diet.
- Improving your diet won't cure chronic constipation, but it is essential to preventing regression and staying healthy in the long run.

CHAPTER 9

WHEN TO CALL IN THE BIG GUNS

M uch of what I have outlined in this book can be implemented by parents and kids independently. That said, some situations call for more direct and personalized interventions. Pediatric physical and occupational therapists who specialize in bowel and bladder issues can be a godsend for certain families. Mental health therapists may be necessary to help heal the parent-child relationship and establish the roles of each family member in treating this condition.

Chapters 4, 5 and 6 provided a general overview of what PTs do to help kids with chronic constipation (and other bowel and bladder challenges). We help build core strength, change breathing patterns, teach posture on the toilet, and work on coordination of the abdominal muscles and pelvic floor muscles when a child is bearing down to have a poop.

So when does your child need skilled PT?

- They can't find a position on the toilet that they can maintain for several minutes, or, their preferred position involves leaning back or leaning far forward so they are touching their toes. Both of these positions make it hard to bear down in an effective way.
- When you ask them to pull up to close the anus, and then bear down to open it, they tell you that they can't feel any movement on their bottom, or they just look at you like you're crazy.
- When you work on "belly big, belly hard" on the toilet, the only way they can make their belly hard is to hold their breath. As soon as they exhale, their belly turns to jelly.
- They generally have lower muscle tone and/or poor coordination. If your kid is always falling on the playground, can't do more than ten jumping jacks in a row before the arms and legs stop moving in sync, or can't stand on one foot for longer than 10 seconds, they might benefit from generalized PT to improve strength and coordination. Even if the therapist is not a pelvic floor specialist, the therapy might have a secondary benefit of improving constipation.

Occupational therapists are a secret weapon in the world of constipation management. Occupational therapists are trained to help people succeed with daily activities. Pediatric OTs help kids learn how to take care of themselves (brush teeth, get dressed), play well with peers, eat a variety of foods, tolerate and work through distractions, and follow multi-step commands. Although only a few OTs are specifically trained in treating pediatric constipation, many pediatric OTs have a variety of skills to help with this issue.

- Picky eating: Picky eating can be due to behavioral issues and anxiety around food, sensitivities to textures and strong tastes, or challenges with oral motor coordination. Depending on the cause, OTs will use different strategies to entice your child to slowly expand what he or she eats. It's not quick or easy, but it does work. It's also enormously important in the long-term management of constipation.

- Sensory processing: Some children under-respond or over-respond to certain stimuli. In day-to-day life, this can mean that a child hates the feel of tags on their clothing or can't focus in a certain type of lighting. In the bathroom, some kids hate the sound of the toilet flushing. Or they have a fear of water splashing up onto their bottom (who doesn't?). Or they are unable to tolerate the silence and stillness required in the bathroom. OTs can assess where a child is over-responsive or under-responsive and help them adjust so they are more successful.

- Interoception: This is a specialized area of OT that can be instrumental in helping kids better manage their constipation. Interoception refers to a person's ability to feel and interpret the sensations happening inside their body. Many kids with chronic constipation have lost the ability to feel the presence of stool in the rectum, if they ever had it. An OT trained in interoception therapy can systematically teach your child how to recognize what they are feeling, and how to act appropriately on that feeling.

- Bathroom routine and hygiene: Occasionally, kids end up with chronic constipation because they are afraid of having a bowel movement in a public restroom or when their parents aren't around. Remember, constipated kids have bowel movements that can be very hard to wipe. Young kids often rely on their parents for help wiping; older kids often make-do, but then end up having a strong odor of poop. If other children tease them because of this odor, they likely will withhold bowel movements during the school day. OTs can help kids learn how to keep themselves clean. They also can help kids learn the bathroom routine. This can be especially useful if kids have cognitive or behavioral challenges that make toileting more difficult.

Finally, a mental health therapist or psychologist may be necessary for your family. By the time you found this book, it's likely you struggled with your child's constipation for quite some time. Even with the best parenting strategies, you may find that you and your child have some issues to work out. I often have parents in tears after they learn what you have learned in this book. They feel terrible for words they said or punishments they implemented. Sometimes the struggle around constipation becomes a generalized power struggle, and parents and kids find themselves clashing over every little thing. Sometimes kids want to give up because they have felt so out of control for so long. If this sounds like your situation, consider getting some mental health support.

To succeed at managing your child's constipation, you and your child are going to have to be on the same page. I've found that a good counselor can help parents and kids find coping strategies to deal with the stress of chronic constipation. The counselor can be a neutral party who helps lay the groundwork for parent-child cooperation rather than conflict. They can also help your child understand that you are trying to help them out of love, not because you are mad at them.

Unless you live in a large urban area or are under the care of a pediatric GI team, you might have a hard time finding a mental health therapist who understands pediatric constipation. That said, I suggest asking your doctor for a list of local child or family counselors or psychologists and calling a few to get a feel for their skills. Questions to ask include:

- Do you have any experience with kids who have chronic constipation? If the therapist does not, give them a brief overview of what you have learned from this book and what areas of constipation management are giving you the most trouble. Hopefully, you'll get a feel for whether the therapist is open to taking on a new type of client.
- My child seems to have anxiety that manifests itself through constipation. How have you helped other children with this issue?
- Have you worked with kids with chronic medical conditions? How have you helped kids who are overwhelmed by all the extra work they need to do for their health that other kids don't seem to need to do?

In the best scenario, you'll find a therapist who is willing to read this book. I have spoken with so many well-intentioned therapists who wrongly assume that most toileting challenges with kids are behavioral unless there is a diagnosed bowel or bladder condition, and that constipation can be treated simply by improving diet. They have all been very receptive to learning more about the physiology behind chronic constipation.

I wrote this book to give you and your child hope. If you and your child commit to the steps I have outlined, I'm confident you will see improvement in your child's constipation and your child will have more energy, appetite and joy after losing the pounds of stool that were weighing them down. I also hope you will see improvement in your whole family's quality of life. Parents who don't constantly feel like they are failing their child because they can't figure out how to get them to poop have more energy to enjoy being parents. Siblings who don't have to change plans all the time because of stomach aches or poop leaks have more time to play together. It will get better!

Wishing you all the best,
Christine Stephenson, PT, DPT
A.K.A. The Constipation Coach

APPENDIX
SECRET SIGNS OF CONSTIPATION

O nce your child has done a clean-out and is receiving a daily laxative dose to keep their stool soft, it can be harder to recognize when they are getting constipated again. At this point, you and your child need to become constipation detectives. If the colon and rectum gradually fill back up, you might lose some of the progress you made with the initial clean-out, and it will take more time to achieve our long-term goal.

Here are some of the "secret signs of constipation". If you notice a few of these symptoms, it might be a good idea to talk to your doctor about doing another clean-out to get back on track.

1) **Poop streaks or hard-to-wipe poops.** Is your child clogging the toilet with toilet paper? Is their underwear always a little bit dirty at the end of the day? Here's the thing: healthy poops, poops that haven't been hanging out in the colon for a long time drying

out, are easy to wipe. Sticky, dry poops are a sign that not all the poop made it out.

2) **Ribbon stools or diarrhea.** If the rectum is full of hard, large stools, the only poop that makes its way out is in the form of ribbons or worms, or, in more serious cases, diarrhea. People often think their child is totally cleaned out when they have diarrhea, when frequently the opposite is true.

3) **Frequent UTIs.** The longer poop hangs out in the rectum, the more bacteria it grows, and, as mentioned above, the harder it is to wipe. This is the same bacteria that causes bladder infections, and it's why chronic UTIs are almost always associated with constipation.

4) **Super stinky, frequent farts.** That bacteria that grows in the rectum? It's stinky. I hear from parents all the time that their child with toileting issues is also the child with the stinkiest farts. I tell kids: a fart is just a poop honking the horn. Toot toot!

5) **Loss of appetite, "grazing" rather than eating a meal, or needing to have a BM in the middle of a meal.** In cases when a kid is super backed up, there is just less room for the stomach to expand to accommodate food.

6) **Wetting the bed.** Constipation is the number one cause of bedwetting. If your child's bedwetting improves after an initial clean-out, but then gradually starts becoming more frequent, you can bet they are getting backed up again.

7) **Your child feels like they have to poop but they can't.** This usually mean that a ball of harder stool has built up in the rectum.

8) **Needing to go pee all the time or waking up at night to pee.** A rectum that is full of poop leaves less room for the bladder to expand. The stool can also press on the bladder, causing it to contract when it doesn't necessarily need to empty.

9) **When your child has to have a bowel movement, they need to have it RIGHT NOW!** Even after a cleanout, the rectum is still stretched out and has decreased sensation. This means that some children only feel poop when they're so full that it's right there at the anus, ready to come out. They run to the bathroom to avoid a leak.

10) **Bellyaches.** The number one cause of stomach aches in kids is constipation. When your child has a stomachache, ask them where it hurts. If it's tender in the lower left or lower right part of the stomach, it's most likely a backup of stool.

11) **Peeing only a trickle.** Sometimes the stool that is backed up in the rectum presses against the urethra, which is the tube that goes from the bladder to the outside of the body. When this happens, kids will feel like they have to pee very badly, but it will only come out as a trickle.

REFERENCES AND RESOURCES

Chapter 1: What is Constipation?

This summary of the research provides a good overview of the definition of functional constipation and the best management practices for primary care providers (physicians):

Rowan-Legg A; Canadian Paediatric Society, Community Paediatrics Committee. Managing functional constipation in children. *Paediatr Child Health.* 2011;16(10):661-670. https://www.ncbi.nlm.nih.gov/pmc/articles/PMC3225480/

Seattle Children's Hospital publishes its clinical protocol for physicians to manage functional constipation. It is a good reference, especially if your provider is hesitant to treat functional constipation aggressively:

https://www.seattlechildrens.org/globalassets/documents/clinics/gi/functional-constipation-clinical-protocol2.pdf

"The Poo in You" is a wonderful video for kids and their grown-ups that explains how functional constipation develops and how it can lead to fecal incontinence. It was created by a nurse practitioner at Colorado Children's

Hospital, with funding from the North American Society for Pediatric Gastroenterology, Hepatology and Nutrition. It can be found on YouTube or at: https://gikids.org/constipation/

The journal Pediatrics published the study "Association of Constipation and Fecal Incontinence With Attention-Deficit/Hyperactivity Disorder" in November 2013. Here's the full reference:
McKeown C, Hisle-Gorman E, Eide M, Gorman GH, Nylund CM. Association of constipation and fecal incontinence with attention-deficit/hyperactivity disorder. Pediatrics. 2013 Nov;132(5):e1210-5. doi: 10.1542/peds.2013-1580. Epub 2013 Oct 21. PMID: 24144702; PMCID: PMC4530301.

Chapter 2: First Step: Medication

I encourage you to work closely with your physician to determine what clean-out approach is best for your child. Here are the hospital protocols that I refer to the most when sending parents back to their primary care provider to get the OK for a clean-out:

Seattle Children's Hospital's protocol is a relatively gentle clean-out that is repeated every other weekend:
https://www.seattlechildrens.org/pdf/PE1071.pdf

Nationwide Children's Hospital publishes a nice bowel cleanout sheet that you can bring to your doctor as an outline. She will be able to fill in the blanks for how much Miralax and how much ExLax to give to your child.
https://www.nationwidechildrens.org/family-resources-education/health-wellness-and-safety-resources/helping-hands/bowel-cleanout

Colorado Children's Hospital has one of the most aggressive clean-outs published on the Web. (It's also fun to read because it's a part of the system's clinical pathway for constipation, so it's what the physicians are using for guidance.) In my experience, many kids improve faster when they start with an aggressive clean-out like this one. But definitely run it by your provider first.

https://www.childrenscolorado.org/globalassets/ healthcare-professionals/clinical-pathways/ed-uc- constipation.pdf

Steve Hodge, MD, has everything you need to know about enema protocols on his website. He is a tireless advocate for the Modified O'Regan Protocol, and his work has improved the lives of many kids with very severe constipation.

https://www.bedwettingandaccidents.com/

Chapter 4: How to Sit

The *Journal Of Clinical Gastroenterology* published a study in March of 2019 on the efficacy of a Defecation Postural Modification Device (DPMD), aka a Squatty Potty. Researchers found that the use of a DPMD—Squatty Potty—decreased straining, increased the sensation of completely emptying the bowels, and decreased the amount of time spent pooping. Here is the complete reference:

Modi RM, Hinton A, Pinkhas D, Groce R, Meyer MM, Balasubramanian G, Levine E, Stanich PP. Implementation of a Defecation Posture Modification Device: Impact on Bowel Movement Patterns in Healthy Subjects. *J Clin Gastroenterol.* 2019 Mar;53(3):216-219. doi: 10.1097/ MCG.0000000000001143. PMID: 30346317; PMCID: PMC6382038.

A study published in Digestive Diseases and Sciences in 2003 found that squatting lowers the time needed to have a bowel movement and decreases straining compared to sitting.

Sikirov D. Comparison of straining during defecation in three positions: results and implications for human health. Dig Dis Sci. 2003 Jul;48(7):1201-5. doi: 10.1023/a:1024180319005. PMID: 12870773.

Chapter 5: Bearing Down

Way back in 1985, researchers from the University of Iowa did quite the study: they inserted water-filled balloons into the rectums of 31 kids, some of whom were constipated, some had encopresis, and some were healthy. They measured muscle activity in the rectum, pelvic floor and anal sphincters while these kids pooped out the balloons. The subjects who were constipated or had fecal incontinence needed to have much more water in the balloons to feel the urge to defecate. They also had difficulty relaxing the pelvic floor while defecating. The researchers concluded that 48% of the constipated subjects had a pelvic floor dysfunction. Here is the full reference:

Loening-Baucke, V., Thompson, R. 694 Pelvic Floor Dysfunction in Children with Chronic Constipation. *Pediatr Res* 19, 226 (1985). https://doi.org/10.1203/00006450-198504000-00724

Chapter 6: How to Move

The Internet has so, so many resources to help families move more. Once you have tired of the exercises in Chapter 6, or if you want to supplement them, go online to find more.

- I really like www.gonoodle.com for younger kids, and for grownups like me who really liked summer camp.

- Jaime, on www.cosmickids.com, is an amazing, fun yoga teacher for younger kids.
- For more serious work-outs, several fitness streaming apps have classes for families to take together. These include Peloton and Obe (with monthly subscriptions after a free trial), and Fitness Blender (with some free classes and content with a subscription).

Here are some IRL (that is: in real life) activities to seek out, too:

- Check out your local YMCA and other gyms for their family options. Our Y offers a family unicycle night throughout the winter and of course family basketball and other racquet sports.
- Call your city's parks department. Usually, they are super happy to talk about activities for families. Our high school track team hosts track meets for elementary kids in the spring.
- Many local organizations host "color runs" during the year, where participants get powdered dye thrown on them while they run. Not my thing, but apparently really fun? In any case, be on the lookout for fun family fitness events that happen close to you throughout the year.

Chapter 7: Stress

Researchers don't know exactly how stress causes constipation, but the connection between the brain and the gut is a huge area of research, and I expect we will know a lot more in coming years.

One large study in Sri Lanka found a higher prevalence of constipation in kids who had undergone stressful events like separation from a best friend, failure of an exam in school, parental job loss, and family member illness. Here's the reference:

Devanarayana NM, Rajindrajith S. Association between constipation and stressful life events in a cohort of Sri Lankan children and adolescents. J Trop Pediatr. 2010 Jun;56(3):144-8. doi: 10.1093/tropej/fmp077. Epub 2009 Aug 20. PMID: 19696192.

Another very large study linked stressful events between the ages of 2.5- to 4-years-old with chronic constipation later in childhood. Interestingly, this study also found that children without a regular sleep routine were almost twice as likely as other children to have chronic constipation.

Joinson, C., Grzeda, M.T., von Gontard, A. *et al.* Psychosocial risks for constipation and soiling in primary school children. *Eur Child Adolesc Psychiatry* 28, 203–210 (2019). https://doi.org/10.1007/s00787-018-1162-8

Two of my favorite resources to help introduce deep breathing and mindfulness to kids (and their grown-ups) are Cosmic Kids Yoga (again) and the Calm app (www. calm.com).

Cosmic Kids Yoga has a series of videos called "Zen Dens" that teach mindfulness and another called "Peace Outs" that are guided relaxation exercises. When browsing videos on the site, sort by "energy" and choose "calm."

The Calm app requires a monthly subscription, but it has been a worthwhile expense for my family and many of my patients. The app has deep breathing and relaxation exercises for every age group. As a bonus, it also has sleep stories for adults and kids that are super effective at calming down the brain when you are trying to achieve an earlier bedtime.

Chapter 8: How to Eat

A very large systematic review published in 2012 found that the studies available at that time were too limited or too contradictory to make any solid recommendation regarding fiber intake. Sometimes increasing dietary fiber helps chronic constipation, sometimes it makes things worse. It might depend on the degree of constipation. It might depend on the way you go about increasing fiber. You can read all about it here:

Maria L Stewart, Natalia M Schroeder, Dietary treatments for childhood constipation: efficacy of dietary fiber and whole grains, *Nutrition Reviews*, Volume 71, Issue 2, 1 February 2013, Pages 98–109, https://doi.org/10.1111/nure.12010

Cow's milk is linked to pediatric functional constipation in this study:

Dehghani SM, Ahmadpour B, Haghighat M, Kashef S, Imanieh MH, Soleimani M. The Role of Cow's Milk Allergy in Pediatric Chronic Constipation: A Randomized Clinical Trial. *Iran J Pediatr*. 2012;22(4):468-474.

... and in this one:

Iacono G, Cavataio F, Montalto G, Florena A, Tumminello M, Soresi M, Notarbartolo A, Carroccio A. Intolerance of cow's milk and chronic constipation in children. *N Engl J Med*. 1998 Oct 15;339(16):1100-4. doi: 10.1056/NEJM199810153391602. PMID: 9770556.

Regarding probiotics, this is the study that reviewed all the published literature on the effectiveness of probiotic supplements:

Gomes DOVS, Morais MB. Gut Microbiota and the Use of Probiotics in Constipation in Children and Adolescents: Systematic Review. *Rev Paul Pediatr*. 2019;38:e2018123. Published 2019 Nov 25. doi:10.1590/1984-0462/2020/38/2018123

Chapter 9: When to get more help

The Herman and Wallace Pelvic Rehabilitation Institute trains many of the physical therapists specialized in pelvic floor rehab. You can find therapists trained by Herman and Wallace on www.pelvicrehab.com.

The Star Institute trains many occupational therapists in sensory processing disorders. You can find a Star-trained OT here: https://www.spdstar.org/treatment-directory.

Kelly Mahler is an occupational therapist who is leading her field in developing and testing therapy to improve a patient's interoception. Currently, the best way to find an interoception-trained OT is to join the "Interoception, the 8th sensory system" group, on Facebook.

ACKNOWLEDGMENTS

My patients and their families were my biggest inspiration when writing this book. It is a big leap of faith to discuss the ins and outs of bowel and bladder challenges with a therapist. My patients put their faith in me, and I tried my best to rise to the challenge.

I would not have embarked down this constipation journey if Robin Lund, a fellow PT, had not invited me to join her and graciously shared all she had learned with me. And that would not have been possible if our employer, LifeScape, had not created the professional space for us to learn and expand our practice into this slightly unusual (at the time) realm. I am forever grateful to Robin and the rest of the LifeScape team.

Dawn Sandalciddi's pediatric course from the Herman and Wallace Pelvic Rehabilitation Institute provided me with the basics of pediatric pelvic floor rehab, and I'm so thankful for her instruction.

So many other friends, colleagues, and referring providers have been a part of this project in one way or another:

brainstorming on how to treat challenging cases, fleshing out the book idea, being an early reader, and making me laugh with poop jokes. I owe a debt of gratitude to all of them, but especially to Megan Trifilo, who just may have given me every good idea I think I've had in the last four years, and to Jen Hasvold, who can somehow shed new light on every subject we discuss.

Eric Abrahamson brings so much more than editing skills to a friendship. But in this instance, I'm grateful for his editing, and for his wife Lois Facer, who is also a gifted reader.

To know my husband Hans is to love him. To live with him is to benefit from his kindness, intelligence, and humor (almost) every day. Also, he is an excellent partner in our other life project: the upbringing of the amazing Elsa and Irene. For all the days when it is "just mom and dad and Elsa and Irene," I am most grateful of all.

ABOUT THE AUTHOR

CHRISTINE STEPHENSON is a physical therapist practicing in Rapid City, South Dakota. She started as a therapist in 2008 and has spent her entire career working with kids. In addition to being a PT, she enjoys running (which she calls her therapy), reading, forcing her kids on hikes, and being forced by them to play Just Dance on the Switch. She also loves to eat, and doesn't mind cleaning the kitchen before, during, and after her husband Hans' culinary adventures.